The Medical Manager

A practical guide for clinicians

Second Edition

Anthony E Young

Guy's and St Thomas' Hospital Trust, St Thomas' Hospital, London, UK

© BMJ Publishing Group 1999, 2003
BMJ Books is an imprint of the BMJ Publishing Group

All rights reserved. No part of this publication may be
reproduced, stored in a retrieval system, or transmitted,
in any form or by any means, electronic, mechanical,
photocopying, recording and/or otherwise, without the prior
written permission of the publishers.

First published in 1999
Second edition 2003
by BMJ Publishing Group, BMA House, Tavistock Square,
London WC1H 9JR

www.bmjbooks.com

British Library Cataloguing in Publication Data

A catalogue record for this book is available from
the British Library

ISBN 0-7279-1781-1

Typeset by SIVA Math Setters, Chennai, India
Printed and bound in Spain by GraphyCems, Navarra

Contents

Preface

We live our lives forwards, we explain them backwards. This book, in part, is the explaining backwards of 12 years spent in medical management; the first four as a Director of Surgical Services, the second four as a Medical Director of Guy's and St Thomas' Hospital Trust and the last four watching from the sidelines to see how others do it. In explaining backwards and advising forwards one's views are bound to be coloured by a set of beliefs, and I admit at the outset a continuing if anxious belief in the NHS as a public service; in the context of an underfunded, poorly directed service it is very effective (as distinct from efficient). However, the NHS has faults for which everyone in it, not just politicians, are partly responsible. Doctors have traditionally played a role in guiding the service in the right direction and helping it to withstand the ill effects of politicisation, underresourcing, and the endless rearrangements that it suffers. Their primacy in this managerial role is no longer as clear as it was, and they need to renew their belief in that role and their skills at achieving it. Hence this book is written for those sceptical about the role of clinicians in management, for doctors in training, and lastly, for those who are freshly into clinical management posts and looking for some "street knowledge".

I hope this book will help those who wish to help guide the service by involving themselves in its day to day management. The text may seem somewhat didactic but that is its purpose for my intention was to make it a practical guide. Much of what I have written I did not know when I first became a medical manager (I wish I had), and most of what I have written has been learnt from experience or I have found that experience has fitted with theory. Where experience has been at variance with what is in the books I have said so. In those disagreements I have not claimed to be the little boy commenting on the emperor's clothes, I have merely noted that the clothes are nowhere near as grand as they are claimed. The little boy of the story was no doubt taken home and soundly spanked, and I expect some of what I have to say will be seen by acolytes of the management revolution as either reprehensible ignorance or an inability to comprehend the true path to the glorious future. That would be sad, as some of the preoccupations of managerialism stand to destroy as much good as they may create.

When I started revising the book for this second edition I had hoped that much of the antimanagerialism that doctors express would have been diluted by familiarity during the five years between editions. The result of the Consultants' Contract ballot in Autumn 2002 and the subsequent recriminations and ill humour showed that little has changed and there is still much to be done.

This is a single-author book so I have perhaps been lopsided in my stress on certain subjects which have concerned me to the neglect of others, which have been less interesting or less problematical. Nevertheless, I hope I have covered the ground across which medical managers exercise their responsibilities. In doing so I have deliberately dwelt on those topics which affect medical managers in their proper role as intermediaries between medicine and management. The territory is necessarily viewed predominantly from an acute hospital perspective, but surveys of medical managers' work shows homogeneous activities, problems, and aspirations across all types of hospital and health authority.

Note on terminology: I have used the term "medical management" at its most general, meaning any form of management with which doctors may become involved. I have used the term "clinical management" to cover the more specific activity of a clinician managing a clinical directorate or team.

Note on references: In trying to avoid references from journals to which most clinicians have no access I have relied heavily on items from the *British Medical Journal* because they are easily accessible in full text form over the internet at bmj.com. Internet references were correct at 1st January 2003.

Note for doctors in training

This is not a textbook of management practice, but you do not need such a textbook any more than a non-clinical manager needs a textbook of medicine. This book is intended to give you a feel for what medical management is about and also contains practical tips for those about to become actively involved. As a trainee looking at the business of management from the outside you may have been confused by the competing passions of the objectors on one side and the management acolytes on the other. It does not matter with which side your natural sympathies lie because the economic and managerial aspects of medical practice are inescapable, so you will need to have a feel for the issues. Very few doctors in the future NHS will find that they can ignore the pressure to become involved in practical managerial tasks and most senior trainees know that the chief executive and medical director of the trust in which they are seeking a consultant job will probably be on the appointments committee. These managers will not unreasonably expect a positive as well as an informed attitude to management issues. May I suggest, therefore, that if you are skimming this book you flit through Chapter 1 then skip to Chapter 3, looking at Sections 3.5, "Managing a budget", 3.6, "Business planning", and 3.7, "Managing for quality", for the important general topics. Section 4.3 in Chapter 4 deals with managing conflict, Section 4.7 is about difficult colleagues, and the whole of Chapter 6 covers the sort of problem areas in which you might be expected to take a view. Lastly, Chapter 5 about the NHS as an institution has some background information which may help you to structure your views of the NHS in the general context of a public service. I hope that at the end of all that you will have enough of a feel for the issues to be able to make your own informed judgments.

Acknowledgments

I would never have thought to write this book if it were not for the stimulating good fellowship of medical, nursing, and managerial colleagues at St Thomas' and at Guy's who stimulated and advised on the first edition and were patient with my awkward questions as the second edition progressed. I am also grateful to all at BMJ Books for their skill and encouragement. Lastly, and above all others, to my wife who in difficult times never wavered in her support during the first edition and without whose encouragement neither edition would ever have been completed.

Anthony E Young

Introduction

Many clinicians hold a sceptical or even frankly negative view of medical management, yet many will wittingly or unwittingly be swept into medical management posts or wish to find out more. Unfortunately, if they look for guidance they may find themselves immediately uncomfortable with the unquestioning faith in managerialism and medical management expressed in most books on the subject. The introductory chapter to one such book is entitled "On the Road to Damascus".[1]

Many doctors harbour a perception that for a clinician to be a manager is to desert his true calling, that clinical management is a disreputable even degrading job, and that the motives for doing it are at best incomprehensible and at worst an exercise in self aggrandisement. I overstate the case, but not by as much as you might think. The reader of books and articles about medical management will find no inkling of the suspicion and anxiety that colours so many clinicians' views; such publications are hallmarked with a halcyon image of a man in a grey suit and a man in a white coat arm in arm with the woman with big shoulder pads striding purposefully into the roseate dawn of the sweetly managed health service. The books contain a wealth of information to help this happy trio carry out their jobs ever better, but almost never do they address the gut feelings of disquiet and frustration felt by most clinicians. These books are predicated on the assumption that the faults in the NHS are due to archaic attitudes and practices within the service and could be solved if only every clinician could be taught to "understand management". By contrast, I hope that this book will address those clinicians' anxieties and the causes for them. I have not replicated the tone of other books on management nor covered the field in the same way. I have dwelt somewhat on the areas most clinicians find difficult, irritating or particularly opaque, and have avoided other purely technical areas where all that would be needed is a reference book. Nevertheless, you should not expect this book to feed all your antimanagerial prejudices or debunk the need for doctors in management. The thesis of this book is simple: firstly, doctors have the aptitude and the knowledge to

Figure 1 The Caduceus. The wings represent transcendence, diligence, and activity. The wand represents power, the axis mundi, down which messages travel between heaven and earth. The double serpents represent the dualist opposites, healing versus poison, illness versus health. They also represent mediation between the upper and lower realms, Good and Evil. Altogether the perfect symbol of office for the medical manager, interlocutor, and healer.

enable them to be managers or to integrate with managers; secondly, they have an obligation to do so as one of the means towards fulfilling their primary task—the proper care of patients, and lastly, they can do so without selling their souls to their imaginary devil. In accepting the need to be involved with or as managers they should nevertheless console themselves with the fact that although much is wrong with the Health Service, much is also wrong with some of the remedies and the way they are administered. Doctors need to help get it right. The interwoven serpents of the physician's symbol, the caduceus, do after all symbolise healing through the balancing of opposing forces (Figure 1).[2]

> We need not fall victim to the liberal fallacy of assuming that because we can perceive a problem we are, *de facto*, not part of the problem.
>
> (David Mamet on "Decay"[3])

References

1 Grime P. On the Road to Damascus. In: Lees P, ed. *Navigating the NHS*. Abingdon: Radcliffe Medical Press, 1996.
2 Cooper JC. *Encyclopedia of Traditional Symbols*. London: Thames and Hudson, 1978.
3 Mamet D. Decay: some thoughts for action. In: *A Whore's Profession*. London: Faber & Faber, 1992, pp 186–92.

1: Doctors as managers

1.1 Management and the profession of medicine

To understand why so many clinicians are dissatisfied and why they focus so much of this dissatisfaction onto managers and the process of management, one needs to look back to see what has been happening over the past 15 years. "Too many managers" is seen simplistically as the problem, when analysis shows it is the *managerialism,* of which they are merely a symptom, that is the true cause of the unhappiness. The core of that managerialism is the presumption that the failings of the National Health Service (NHS) are a result of attitudes and processes that are fundamentally flawed and could be solved by the imposition of a new order by managers. This "new order", this managerialism, is a mix of an obsession with control, accountability and measurement overlaid onto a hotch potch of different business management theories imported into the public sector, historically late and frequently inappropriately. For clinicians as for other professionals the real damage is done by the consequential lack of professional autonomy which denies their *professionalism* and goes cheek by jowl with a progressive loss of *power.* It is not easy to separate loss of professionalism from loss of power, but would-be managers need to understand clinicians' views about this erosion of status. They also need to understand how the new finance- and performance-based managerialism may damage the public service values of the people it affects, leading to a deterioration in morale and performance which overshadows the benefits that are supposed to accrue. Private sector management theory is not transportable to public services without major modification.[1] Doctors can and should be involved in the management of the NHS at all levels, for they are the most appropriate group for the task. Why? A crude summary of Luke's thesis of the three dimensions of power[2] identifies them as:

- controlling the agenda
- controlling expectations
- controlling the players.

The dominance of the medical profession in each of these areas shrinks daily but is still predominant. I know that most managers would say that doctors have an inappropriately powerful stranglehold on the delivery of health care, and find it difficult to understand clinicians' anxieties. They may not perceive how the culture of managerialism is insidiously taking over territory previously solely within the clinician's demesne and even in quite small details denying their power to judge what process of care is best for patients. This is not a phenomenon solely experienced by doctors but is simply an expression of a wider trend in society as the power, status and privileges of the professions are eroded. Within the NHS some territorial incursions are inadvertent, such as changes to the processes of appointment and rotation of junior staff, and the way beds are now managed. These changes with many others can mean that clinicians no longer feel that they have an accountable staff and a defined physical territory and are increasingly uncertain about their prerogatives, even when face to face with patients. When combined with covert and indeed overt messages that doctors cannot be trusted to run the business of healthcare it all contributes to the demoralisation that can lead to poor performance at one end of the scale or bolshie confrontationalism at the other. At the very least it feeds the antimanagerial culture prevalent among clinicians—70% of doctors are reported as antipathetic to managers. In exploring this further the cherished notion of clinicians' professionalism is itself worth exploring.

Professionalism and its erosion

We need to understand what we mean when as doctors we describe ourselves as *professionals*. At its simplest we imply an exclusive, collegiate grouping, defining and administering a set of skills. It is a social as much as a technical phenomenon, but a profession derives its power from those skills, unlike bureaucrats who derive power primarily from their position. For doctors professionalism goes far beyond the collegiate for doctors tend to admit only one view of their professional ethos, the humanistic, caring view, and indeed it is important that they do so for there are other opinions which identify our professionalism as simply an exercise in self interest or just as an unhelpful social phenomenon. But more of this later;

first to flesh out the traditional view, the average doctor's self image.

The doctors' view of professionalism

NHS doctors do not accept that they are working "under" anyone outside the profession, only within the managerial framework of a public service and the professional constraints laid on them by the General Medical Council; they work for patients.

(Lee Potter)[3]

Within the ambit of one's professionalism as a clinician one might properly claim to know about disease and its treatment, and about what patients need and want; but one quite reasonably might also claim to know how best to define and deliver the services which affect those patients and their illnesses. Also, one could claim some primacy in knowing how best to educate and choose one's successors. The margins of all these areas are being nibbled away. There is a hazier area concerning professionalism which is to do with personal conduct and the emotional and physical commitment that doctors make to patients. By claiming with nurses sole occupancy of this high ground some doctors are encouraged to believe that there is an automatic rightness in their judgment which cannot be questioned by others; an inheritance of moral authority somewhat akin to priestship. It is this sense of primary responsibility in certain areas of medicine that motivates clinicians. Training, education, experience, and character are perceived as the mainsprings of proper care for patients, as validating the doctor's leadership of the team and giving the right to define the shape of the future of medicine. With a few notable exceptions doctors tend to view this congruent set of skills, activities, and privileges as uniquely theirs. These are indeed the components of their professionalism. Autonomy is a crucial element in this because the relationship between patients or clients and professionals is characterised by patients' minimal or absent knowledge about their problems and their need to enter into a dependent relationship with the doctor. In order to provide an environment in which this trust is not exploited, professionals must be able to act free from outside interference and they must also be free to regulate their profession to protect it from charlatans and the incompetent, and must do so vigorously. Lastly, where there is a team dealing with clinical matters they assert a right to lead that team. Trust is a crucial component of this equation, the patient, the doctor, and the NHS as a public body must all trust each other yet that trust is perceived as being under continuing erosion with very little reason, as Onora O'Neill spelt out in her Reith Lectures of 2002.[4] The alternative to professionalism is centrally directed micromanagement of clinical work by protocol and by contracts. Additionally, lack of trust provides an excuse for government to get rid of those other pillars of professionalism, self regulation and certification, that is, the privilege of defining and controlling the processes of education and examination.

Managers' professionalism

Non-medical managers also perceive themselves as professionals but, by contrast, they see themselves as having universal skills in organisation, finance, planning, people, education. Not unreasonably, they are trained to believe that these skills are portable and that most managers are totipotent, as applicable in a hospital as in a bank or a business. They do not demand autonomy; indeed, they can only exist of part of an hierarchical system of interdependent teams.

When the managers' area of influence overlaps with that of doctors there is bound to be trouble. From the clinician's point of view the overlap was not originally overlap but simply juxtaposition, which was when *managers* were *administrators*— passive implementers of a static set of operational arrangements and clearly lower in the pecking order than doctors. But managers do not want to be administrators, they want to be managers. They hate the term "administrator" and, indeed, to call a manager an administrator is the quickest and most predictable way to annoy. Real managers want to make things happen differently. They live by change and for change. If nothing changes they do indeed simply become administrators (in effect they usually just leave). Change is the engine, the tonic, the aphrodisiac, and as we are living in an era of continuous change in medicine, the manager quickly becomes a major player on a level with the clinician. Change is not perceived by clinicians as central to their life in medicine.

Change is not a feature of the core activity: cancers are still cut out; diabetes is still treated with insulin; fractures plastered; and leaky valves replaced.

When managerialism first began to intrude into clinical practice it was into those areas at the edge of the medical empire where the clinician's hold is less confident—the organisation of care delivery, priority setting, education, finance. Most recently the incursions have become bolder and will become more so as legislative changes have made the manager also directly responsible for service quality; this *de facto* involves them in the details of clinical practice. What troubles doctors is not so much the fact of change as the details of change and the reality that change is predominantly commissioned and led at all levels by non-doctors and, furthermore, that those non-doctors are increasingly questioning how doctors do things.

If you wish to assess the effect this is having on doctors simply look around you, read the non-clinical parts of the journals, the letters columns, talk to doctors and managers and ask how many clinicians have planned early retirement. A BMA survey of 800 doctors in April 1996 found that seven out of ten suffered from work-related stress and 88% considered they were more stressed than they had been five years earlier. Of those reporting work-related stress, more than 25% had increased their alcohol intake to help them cope and one in five had contemplated suicide.[5] Another study found that whereas increasing seniority was previously associated with less stress that now seems to be reversed, higher stress levels being reported in consultants than house officers.[6] A separate and more scientific assessment by Ramirez and colleagues also reported high stress levels and identified the top three causes of stress as work overload, feeling poorly managed and resourced and, lastly, the impact of managerial responsibilities. Nevertheless these authors confirmed that "the transfer of various responsibilities from clinicians to managers may undermine professional morale".[7] Another study has shown that two-thirds of general practice principals had considered leaving general practice, the commonest reason being "increasing bureaucracy/government interference".[8] And do not think it is just the old fogies too sclerotic to accept healthy change. Isobel Allen, of the Policies Studies Institute, studied the "core values" of doctors aged under 40 ("Committed but Critical"). Her conclusion was that young doctors are developing a widespread sense of isolation and alienation caused chiefly by the managerial culture within the NHS. Other research by the Policy Studies Institute has shown a worrying acceleration in the number of young doctors who regret their decision to study medicine, a rise from 26% of male graduates in 1976 to 58% of 1986 graduates and, appallingly, a rise from 30% for 1976 female graduates to 76% for the 1986 cohort.[9] Many stresses account for this but many are in the areas encompassed by managerialism and deprofessionalisation. My own survey of the reasons why clinicians plan to retire early found deprofessionalisation, bureaucracy, overregulation and pressures imposed by managers to be the biggest causes of wishing to leave, second only to the pressure of on-call work.[10]

The focal point of clinicians' professionalism is an assumed right of pre-eminence in defining what is the correct and incorrect treatment for illnesses, and all their powers flow from that. However, even at this centre point of medical professionalism clinicians' primacy is being challenged by managers empowered by evidence-based medicine, emboldened by holding the budget or the power to define a contract. Once that core area in clinical professionalism is invaded by others, clinicians potentially become mere technologists, creatures of protocols and service specifications. The continued sniping by politicians and the media, and the latter's ill-informed promotion of alternative medicine, adds to the overall feeling of a profession under threat. Crucially, there is also a self-destructive effect from the widespread cynicism that infuses clinicians' interpretation of most management-driven reforms. Normally announced as improvements in quality or quantity of service for patients, clinicians still perceive these usually as concealed attempts at cost savings or as the populism of politicians. All this sounds very unhappy, very unsatisfactory and clearly needs to be addressed. Indeed, this is the true crisis in the NHS. Deprofessionalisation is the germ that has infected the system and has the power progressively to devitalise it. The rejection in 2002 of a proposed new contract by consultants and overwhelmingly by trainees was symptomatic of this trend. We really have not moved on from where we were in 1990 when Klein wrote:

> Given the certainty that conflict will continue and the possibility that the NHS may be living off an inherited but not necessarily renewable

capital of commitment and loyalty is it possible to devise better strategies for managing the resentment generated by mutual dependency of the state and the profession?[11]

What are we to do then?

Redefining professionalism

Clinicians (doctors who touch patients) must redefine their professionalism and incorporate in the new definition a concept of understanding citizenship as well as individualism. Additionally they will need to embrace the management of change and be able to manage that change effectively and constructively. They will need to learn to work humbly in teams and accept that others besides doctors have valid views about how best to provide medical care. They will need to share with non-clinical managers those marginal areas mentioned earlier and to regard the contributions of those managers as potentially constructive rather than solely destructive. To do so they are going to have to learn to be effective in those areas themselves, and most are going to have to become managers in one form or another while still being doctors. The paradox and the irony of this is that redemption from their anxieties about managers lies in becoming one. On the other side of the divide the government, health authorities, public health doctors and non-clinical managers are going to have to learn the difference between a doctor and a manager and are going to have to modulate their enthusiasm for change for the sake of change and understand that significant and real autonomy is the key to getting the best out of professionals. If doctors are not faced by successive waves of inappropriate change and inappropriate populist dictats and obsessional central control they may be able to adjust to the new environment, redefine their professionalism and regain their morale; possibly even their primacy in the system. It is a lesson of history as well as of biology that success comes only through adaptation.

Other interpretations of medical professionalism

In the 1960s and 1970s the much quoted *Medical Nemesis* by Ivan Illich[12] centred on the claim that the profession and science of medicine far from improving the health of society, was in fact, superfluous. That view is no longer fashionable nor scientifically tenable, but clinicians should be aware of two other interpretations of medical professionalism which social scientists like to air.

The first might be called the "Monopolistic Control" view.

> It is argued that professionals ... actually act in pursuit of self interest rather than client/patient interest. Thus the characteristics of professionalism such as autonomy and self regulation help to produce a situation in which managerial control and supervision can be evaded, and in which the practice of specific skills can be retained as a monopoly within the profession, helping keep earnings higher, and career prospects better than would otherwise have been the case.[13]

This fits well with the simplistic tenet of "Rational Choice theory", which was fashionable with social scientists in the 1980s—all rational choices are informed only by "knavish" self interest and that financial gain is at its heart. This in turn harmonises with the modern tenets of individualism and belief in the pervasive powers of "the market". Fortunately for those who believe altruism is alive and well, subsequent "research" has cast doubt on this most cynical of theories.

The second might be termed a "neo-Marxist" view and identifies the habits of medical professionalism as secondary to social conditioning. Doctors are selected mainly from middle class backgrounds and are educated within a social elite, they thus take on traditional authority values and continue to reinforce them throughout their careers.[14] Nurses have accepted and mimicked this hierarchical arrangement and patients are conditioned socially to accept it uncritically as an advantageous norm. Furthermore, the ills of society are "medicalised" so that they become "attributes of individuals, not of society as a whole. The hospital becomes symbolic of this as well as of the social power of the medical and nursing professions.[15] Lastly, the political embarrassment of diseases, whether caused by the social structure of the state or unresolved because of rationing or inequitable access, is concealed and mollified by an acquiescent medical profession acting as an agent of the state.[16]

You should know about these alternative and often deeply cynical views of your behaviour, if only because you may find them used to rationalise power struggles or salve the consciences of those who wish to diminish the status of the medical profession. You might also note a not infrequent whiff of class war sentiment in some of what is written about the management of health care; an unadmitted, unconstructive undercurrent.

1.2 Doctors and managers—two tribes?

It has been said that "management is an activity, not a social group", but managers within the NHS are an identifiable separate group of people. If you take on a management role you remain a doctor, yet in some ways you will need to transform into a manager, a different profession with different skills addressing a different type of problem using different styles and methods for dealing with them. To some extent you will be play-acting for as long as you are managing. Professional managers will know this and your relationship with them may be a fruitful journey of mutual support and education, or it may be an unhappy paranoid relationship from which, in due course, you both are relieved to escape. In my experience several issues can sour the relationship. Perhaps the most common occur when newly appointed clinical directors thinks they can breeze into management and be totipotent and effective from the first day: hiring and firing; spending and cutting. This is rarely so. Secondly, new clinical directors may constantly behave as if they are not really part of the management team, feeling able to swing in and out, support or resist initiatives as mood or expediency takes them. These habits are likely to irritate less well paid but just as hard working and professional managers. Conversely, the management tribe may upset doctors in management by expecting them to "come across", leaving behind all their clinician's reflexes and sensitivities. There is no reason why clinicians should not become perfectly good managers without the need for total cultural assimilation. The clinician–manager relationship need not be a *folie a deux* in which both can only coexist because they support the others' delusions. Clinicians need to learn the language of management and to work with managers but not to parody them. Managers and doctors do after all largely share the same objectives and perhaps also the same character attributes which have been identified for doctors by John Butterfield:

- courage
- intelligence
- wisdom
- style

to which I would add

- optimism.

For all this, doctors and managers remain two separate tribes and it does not help to demand that they are the same. The following lists caricature some of the differences.

Doctors	Managers
Moral absolutists	Moral relativists
Deal in specifics	Deal in the general
Autonomous decision taker	Group decision taker
Conservative, suspicious of change	Thrive on change
Scientific	Non-scientific
Long stay in post	Short stay in post

Intellectual equivalence?

The process of medical decision taking is relatively straightforward. There is one patient at a time to consider, using a body of evidence obtained from examining and investigating the patient. That evidence has to be weighed and sifted according to doctors' knowledge and experience, and a management (note the word!) decision made by doctors using all their experience and knowledge, finally modulated by a humanitarian view of this particular patient's needs. Then on to the next patient. Medicine's problems come in neat packages called patients and they can be dealt with quite quickly and one at a time. It is a little difficult, therefore, to understand why clinicians can be so arrogantly dismissive of the intellectual skills of other forms of management. Many of the problems that managers grapple with are more complex, more difficult to analyse, less easily soluble by formula, and carry the added difficulty that implementation of the management plan requires more stamina and greater use of interpersonal skills than is ever called upon in the clinical context.

Moral relativism

This high-sounding phrase identifies a crucial difference between managers and clinicians, an inherent difference which cannot be made to go away by debate. The difference is a factor in the discomfort many clinicians feel about being in managerial posts. At its simplest clinicians believe they are the servant of a set of moral absolutes concerning the care of patients. They maintain an idealised view of their relationship with patients, a sort of heroic one-to-one relationship unsullied by commerce, error or the vagaries of human communication. For example, clinicians may believe that every patient is entitled to every jot of treatment that might be available, that the treatment should be available promptly, and that the length of stay in hospital should be governed only by the true social, personal and medical needs of the patient. There are no such absolutes for the relativist manager, nor can there be. Relativist managers must work within limited resources and cut their cloth appropriately, they must work in a landscape of continuous change and uncertainty. Clinicians increasingly accept the reality of this situation but it does not mean that they like it, and they may believe that to espouse it formally by taking up a management post will run counter to their professional commitment to provide the best available care for all patients. They also identify another argument beyond the simple adherence to a finite budget for they are rightly anxious that as managers they may be put in a position where they must implement policies that are the product not of economics but of political ideology or whim which may work against a patient's true needs. One can share managers' irritation at the overstatement of the moral case that some doctors make. There are too many doctors who seem to be happy to spend their time picnicking on the moral high ground, simply chucking stones at those toiling on the lower slopes trying to raise the staple crop. Nevertheless, all need to admit that there is a real and irreconcilable difference of emphasis ... which is actually useful.

Nor should doctors complain at the appearance on the scene of so many managers. In 1981, when Sir Roy Griffiths was collecting evidence for his report on NHS management, doctors were not slow to point out how undermanaged as well as ineptly managed the NHS was. They observed that there seemed to be few effective mechanisms for getting things done. This indeed was the thrust of Griffiths' final report.[17] In his oft-quoted summary of the situation Roy Griffiths said, "if Florence Nightingale were carrying her lamp through the corridors of the NHS today she would almost certainly be searching for the people in charge". That report ended a period of formal consensus management in the NHS and heralded the 18 000 rise in the number of NHS managers between 1989 and 1994 and an increase in the managerial pay bill over the same period from £158·8 million to £723·3 million. Since then the number of "senior managers" has increased by 48% and the overall number of managers by 24%. By 2002 the number of "managers" (including clerks and administrators) was said to exceed the number of beds with a ratio of eight managers to ten nurses. In the private sector by comparison the ratio is said to be two managers to ten nurses. "Nowadays you can't shine your lamp into any part of the organisation without revealing a crowd of people who are supposed to be in charge".[18] It is worth noting though that Griffiths foresaw the need for doctors in managerial posts, and holding and being specifically responsible for budgets.

Lastly, one should be insightful and frank about the negative attitudes that many clinicians have to change or novelty and how they have let go of the helm during the last 15 difficult years of the NHS, allowing initiatives to be shaped by politicians, academic social scientists, economists and managers. We must not be surprised at this, nor prepared to tolerate it. Jeremy Lee-Potter, erstwhile Chairman of the BMA wrote:

> The window dressing from ministers about involving doctors in management is largely tinsel. Lions led by donkeys have a habit of eating the donkeys in the end![19]

The solution for the lions is to lead and not to be led. An appetite for donkey flesh, however, is not to be discouraged.

References

1 Mintzberg M. *The Rise and Fall of Strategic Planning.* Hemel Hempstead: Prentice Hall, 1994.
2 Luke S. *Power. A Radical View.* London: Macmillan, 1974.
3 Lee-Potter J. *A Damn Bad Business.* London: Gollancz, 1997.
4 O'Neill O. *A Question of Trust.* Cambridge: CUP, 2002.
5 Coulson J. Doctors under stress. *BMA News Rev* 1996;April:22–6.
6 Karpur N, Borrill C, Stride C. Psychological morbidity and job satisfaction in hospital consultants and junior house officers. *BMJ* 1998;**317**:511–12.
7 Ramirez AJ *et al.* Mental health of hospital consultants: the effects of stress and job satisfaction at work. *Lancet* 1996;**347**:724–8.
8 Spurgeon P, Barwell F, Maxwell R. Types of work stress and the implications for the role of general practitioners. *Health Serv Management Res* 1995;**8**:186–97.
9 Allen I. *Doctors and their Careers.* London: Policy Studies Institute, 1994, p. 229.
10 Young AE. Why consultants take early retirement. *Bull R Coll Surg Engl* 2002;**84**:230–2.
11 Klein R. The State and the profession: the politics of the double bed. *BMJ* 1990;**301**:700.
12 Illich I. *Medical Nemesis: the Expropriation of Health.* London: Calder and Boyars, 1975.
13 Harrison R, Pollitt C. *Controlling Health Professionals.* Milton Keynes: Open University Press, 1994, pp 2–3.
14 Hadley R, Forster D, eds. *Doctors as Managers.* London: Longman, 1986, p. 162 *et seq.*
15 Friedson E. *Profession of Medicine: a Study of the Sociology of Applied Knowledge.* London: Harper & Row, 1970.
16 Turner BS. *Medical Power and Social Knowledge.* London: Sage, 1987, chap. 7.
17 Griffiths Sir R. *Report of the NHS Management Enquiry.* London: DHSS, 1983.
18 Micklethwait J, Wooldridge A. *The Witch Doctors.* London: Mandarin, 1997, p. 341.
19 Lee-Potter J. *A Damn Bad Business.* London: Gollancz, 1997, p. 242.

2: Starting up as a medical manager

Before you accept a medical management post there are questions to ask yourself:

- Do I want to do it and why?
- Am I the right age?
- What will the job involve?
- Do I have the necessary skills?
- How do I prepare myself?

2.1 Do I want to do it?

We can subdivide this question into four:

- Do I want to do it as an end in itself?
- Or as a means to an end?
- Or as a simple professional obligation, or
- Because I have been dragooned or flattered into it?

Few people enter medical management because they wish it to be the main focus of the rest of their professional lives, and I suspect that most do so simply because they feel they ought to. They do not do it resentfully and the prospect will probably interest them. By contrast, it is worth mentioning that there are some disreputable reasons for going in as well, which may help you in making your decision. For example, "I don't want anyone else to do the job", "I don't believe anyone can do the job as well as I can", "I want to have power over my colleagues", or, "I want to use it as a vehicle to get what I want from the organisation". Alternatively, perhaps you are a "control freak"—a much overused term which I take to mean that you need to have a finger in every pie, to have everything possible under your control. You must not be under any illusion that it will make you popular. In this context you can bear in mind the Congolese proverb "the higher up the tree the monkey climbs the more his bottom shows" or more politely quote yourself St Luke, "It needs must be that offences come, but woe unto those through whom they come". Lastly, do not expect to do it to make money. It may increase your salary a bit and if you do it well it just might help you in the distinction award stakes, but rarely enough to offset the hassles.

You will need to have a moderately rounded personality, for the successful manager needs a diversity of traits and skills if the job is to be done adequately—interpersonal skills of course, an ability to collate and react to information, the ability to plan and to implement the plan. I must confess to enjoying planning but like much less the hard grind of execution. I have discovered that this is not merely my problem, it is widespread, and managers often enjoy the planning which should be 10% of the effort but are much less enthralled by the other 90% of effort that needs next to be expended on execution.

2.2 Am I the right age?

The correct age for appointment to a clinical management post is often debated and there is no right answer. It is, however, good practice for young clinicians to look at their possible future career path before accepting a management post. Clinical director posts are time consuming and reduce the opportunities for developing or practising other skills. Furthermore, when clinicians have spent a few years in management posts they have learnt a set of skills and obtained a body of knowledge that makes them very valuable assets to the organisation ... but only if they continue in management. As a consequence, some young clinicians become "trapped" into a sequence of management posts from which they may emerge too late to develop other, possibly more rewarding, avenues of personal development. We need young clinicians in management for their vigour, open mindedness and longevity, but the potential damage to the full breadth of an individual's career needs to be considered and discussed openly before appointment. Senior jobs, such as medical directors and executive committee members, may be more appropriate for older, more streetwise clinicians. The actual ages of 702 clinical directors who responded to a British

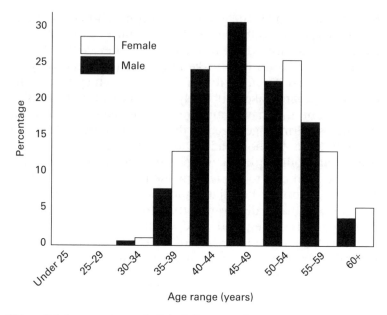

Figure 2.1 Age spectrum of clinical directors. (Data source: British Association of Medical Managers, 1997.)

Association of Medical Managers (BAMM) survey is shown in Figure 2.1. Newly appointed consultants must be very wary of invitations to be clinical directors made before they have barely had time to hang up their coats on day one! Such an invitation implies a problem with the team they have just been asked to manage; problems which combined with a lack of experience of the unit may make the job singularly difficult if they are fool enough to accept there and then. Wait!

2.3 Do I have the skills?

You certainly must not think that because you were intelligent and laborious enough to qualify as a doctor that you can automatically slip into management and be good at it. Also you must not think that because your clinical firm works well you thereby have the skills needed to run a more complex business with a less well-defined hierarchy.

In so far as personal qualities are concerned you will be helped by having:

- *patience*—which includes tolerating long waits to see things happen
- *resilience*—willingness to put up with repeated frustrations
- *perspicacity*—the ability to see the wood despite the trees
- *leadership skills.*

You will also need some practical skills, chief among which I would include the following.

- The ability to read amounts of exceptionally boring paperwork at times when you are tired and yet be able to extract the crucial facts from it.
- The ability to understand the work and attitudes of people not normally in your ambit.
- Time management—I have to confess that this was something I personally never managed, indeed I even failed to find the time to attend the one-day time management course which had been booked for me.

Leadership skills

Leadership is something that you *do* rather than something that you *are,* yet I suspect most people believe that leaders are born and not made and that, furthermore, charismatic heroes existed in history. They might therefore believe that in smaller environments there must be those imbued with smaller versions of these skills of leadership and equally those that are bereft of them. Historians have searched for the skills that mark out great leaders from other mortals and no biography is complete without that sort of analysis, but the skills do not seem to be common between leaders. Modern social science fashion takes the antiheroic view that leadership depends more on context and is dependent on the character of the followers and the particular situation to hand rather than to any special powers that a leader might have. Churchill, for example, was an excellent wartime leader but an unremarkable peacetime leader. Leadership in the powerful, directive sense is simply unfashionable in this age of passive liberalism. The autonomy of little groups is considered to be the mainspring of productive work and they need to be "facilitated" rather than directed. The age of the intermediary is indeed upon us[1] and the manager has become the true intermediary, functioning primarily as a catalyst. For medical managers this is important because fashionably their leadership is supposed to be through quiet influencing rather than through rabble-rousing oratory or a publicly glamorous leadership persona. Leadership will need to be through example, particularly in the style of their clinical performance. However persuasive a medical manager's tongue, it is unlikely that colleagues will be persuaded to accept a rule or a change if he or she fails openly to accept them. Leadership is, after all, a mutual relationship between the leader and the led, in which leaders must balance three crucial components: The Task ... The Team ... and The Individual. In so doing, leaders need WIST (Wisdom, Integrity, Sensitivity and Tenacity).[2]

Despite this seeming absence of overt leadership characteristics, someone will no doubt have spotted some old-fashioned leadership skills in you before offering you a management job, so you do not need to be on the lookout for a course or a book on leadership skills—you may already have them. In 1513 Machiavelli, the first management guru, wrote *The Prince* as a leadership course for Duke Lorenzo the Magnificent of Florence, but the Duke felt it was unnecessary for someone already confidently in post, preferring a pair of hunting dogs given to him at the same time by another suitor. He would probably have supported Lord Sheppard's view of leadership as "Management by a light grip on the throat".

Incidentally, I believe we do have some need for heroic leaders in the NHS, for grey is indeed the colour of management, and management is not the same as leadership. The red heat of conflict and the purple of passion are not currently welcomed in NHS managers—perhaps they should be. There should be in the NHS what Peters[3] describes as "preachers of vision".[4] Their moment will return because today's truths of management theory are quickly supplanted by those of tomorrow or even yesterday, because one of the features of this sort of social science is that there are no testable truths so your guess about how best to manage is probably as good as theirs, or mine.

2.4 What does it involve? How will I prepare myself?

Too many people enter medical management without a very clear idea of what will be asked of them and therefore not knowing whether they can deliver effectively. Some homework is therefore needed before accepting a medical manager's job. The next chapter outlines what it is that medical managers do, but you will need to make sure that your particular job is defined before you accept it. If you read no other section of this book I would suggest that this is the crucial bit.

You need to be happy that five areas have been dealt with:

- that you have an explicit role
- that you have an explicit contract
- that explicit training is available
- that explicit clinical back-up arrangements have been made
- that explicit arrangements have been made for re-entry into the clinical world at end of the job.

The key word you will have noted is "EXPLICIT".

An explicit role

Ask the following questions.

- What area will I be managing?
- What managerial support will I have?
- What will be my relationship to the managerial support?
- Do they work for me or do I work for them?
- What office support will be available? Check that the extra work will not merely devolve onto your already overloaded clinical secretary.
- What will be my relationship with nursing staff? Is there a nurse manager and what is our professional relationship?
- What are my reporting lines? Am I answerable directly to the chief executive, to the medical director, or to some other medical or non-medical manager?

You should make sure that you have answers to all questions these in the form of a letter, or at very least you should write them down after the first meeting to discuss the job. Clinical directors and medical directors should have explicit job descriptions, though in our Trust we have tried to move away from the convoluted, detailed job description to a more general one. The type of tasks that medical managers undertake are implicit in the contents of this book but more explicit in Sections 3.1 and 4.9.

An explicit contract

More questions to ask.

- How many notional half days am I expected to work at this?
- On an old-style contract will they count as fixed or unfixed sessions? In a new style contract what will they replace?
- What is the term of my job?
- What notice should I give or can I be given?
- What is the remuneration? Is this an honorarium or is it superannuable?
- Is there access to a budget for training and for professional travel?
- Will I be expected to sign a confidentiality clause? Most doctors find such clauses to be an anathema and most would probably refuse to sign one, they are in most instances illegal anyway. They should not be necessary. If your Trust demands one in your contract, make sure that it applies only to genuinely "commercial" issues and not to professional judgments you might make about the care patients are receiving.
- If my sessions are to be *added* to my current NHS sessions and so bring them up to full time or more than full time, will I still be entitled to undertake private practice if I wish?
- What is my budget, who sets it and who reviews it?
- Is there performance related payment (PRP)?

Explicit training

Whether you need any training before taking up your appointment really depends on you and your experience. It is difficult to know which of your skills will be deficient when it comes to management. Many clinical directors have come into post and functioned excellently with no prior management training whatsoever. Membership of the British Association of Medical Managers (BAMM) and, if you are a medical director, the Association of Trust Medical Directors (ATMD) is, I would say, mandatory and attendance at their conferences or some of their short courses would probably suffice for most people. I would like to think that the skills required of a good manager are human skills, quickly learnt by intelligent, open-minded clinicians. If there is formal training which is needed it is about the mechanics of management within the NHS: how the finances work; how decisions are made; how purchasing is undertaken; and so forth. These are listed in Section 4.9 "Professional and personal development". I have an aversion to formal training in management skills, but I must be in a minority because this is a boom industry in the NHS, as elsewhere. Courses in management training, seminars on current issues and mini-conferences abound. As a medical director I received between five and ten announcements for such events in my mail each week, most with glossy, persuasive blurbs puffed out with pictures of the lecturers and selected quotes from contented attenders at previous courses. The common feature of the courses seem to be that one has never heard of 90% of the speakers, 90% are more expensive than seems reasonable on any judgment, 90% have been set up for purely commercial reasons, and 90% of the content of each course seems to be of no immediate relevance to one's real job. As a consequence I quickly reached the point where 90% of such announcements went straight into my wastepaper basket. Reading the pundits you would think that educational information about practical management skills was something new. Anyone who believes that should perhaps read for example the *Meditations* of Marcus Aurelius, written in the second century AD; for example, book VI number 50:

> try to move men by persuasion not against their will if the principles of justice so direct. But if someone uses force to obstruct you, then take a different line; resign yourself without a pang and turn the obstacle into an opportunity for the exercise in some other virtue.

The NHS has an unfortunate habit of trying to mimic today what happened in business the day before yesterday. The present obsession with business management courses is symptomatic of this, although their relevance and effectiveness within the NHS remains untested. Nevertheless, fashion dictates that sending new clinical directors to an expensive country hotel to role play and put up tents blindfold will make things better.

The sceptic will note that the motive for "sending clinicians off on a management course" is frequently not a desire to make them good, practical managers but to inculcate in them an understanding of what managers have to do, and why they have to do it. It is hoped that afterwards they will be more cooperative, or at least sympathetic. That, of course, is an entirely proper motive but it is probably more sensible to start working towards that particular educational objective at the undergraduate stage, though very discreetly.

Although you may not need any formal training, you will certainly need to set aside time for a formal period of induction in which you spend some time with the major players in the organisation generally and in your own area in particular. You must also visit in person each ward, office, outpatient clinic, etc for which you will have responsibility and ensure that the staff there know your name and your face. It is extraordinary how bad doctors are at arranging such induction sessions—usually pleading shortage of time. This induction period is too important to skimp, and it may save you a lot of time later, also it is a good introduction to the skill of "Management By Walking Around" (MBWA).

Books on management theory and the MBA

Bookshops, especially those at airports and stations, have large sections devoted to books about management: *The Way to Win, Think and Grow Rich, The Foundations of Corporate Success, A Passion for Excellence, The One Minute Manager,* and so on, including helpful titles such as *Who Moved my Cheese?* About $750 million worth of books about business is sold every year in the USA alone, and Americans are less addicted to them than the British. Many of these titles have made their authors into millionaires, but it is claimed very few are read from end to end. Managers' anxiety not to be outflanked by a new idea continues to sell these books, whereas faddism and a lack of objective ways of judging their worth guarantees a steady flow of new books. If you are minded to buy one first see if you can get hold of a copy of *The Witch Doctors*,[5] by Micklethwait and Wooldridge. The authors, editors of *The Economist,* appraised all the management gurus' texts and presented the case both for and against them. They summarised the general case against management theorising thus:

- it is constitutionally incapable of self criticism
- its terminology usually confuses rather than educates
- it rarely rises above common sense
- it is faddish and bedevilled by contradictions that would not be allowed in more rigorous disciplines.

That said, these books sometimes make interesting reading when you have a particular problem to hand, but are usually only worth dipping into. What you must not do is believe them. The bestselling management book, *In Search of Excellence*, by Peters and Waterman[6] analysed the factors that led to the success of a cohort of American businesses and exhorted others to copy them. Unfortunately, almost all of those top companies have now fallen from grace. You will probably find something more sustaining elsewhere in the bookshop. If you are in London a trip to the library of the King's Fund in Cavendish Square will allow a look at current textbooks and reports as well as the full range of management journals.

The MBA (Master of Business Administration) is sometimes floated past clinical managers as a "good thing to do". I really think it is inappropriate unless you have quite considerable experience in clinical management and envisage your future in it. Even then it may be a waste of time, the MBA is after all sometimes lampooned by senior managers as "MBA, Maybe Best Avoided". In the USA nearly 100 000 MBAs are awarded each year. In the UK, currently, 100 institutions offer MBAs and the part-time courses last between two and five years. They are expensive, part-time courses costing from £10 000 to £15 000 and even up to £30 000, though to be fair the expensive one does include the cost of meals.[7] These courses place enormous pressure on participants to devote their spare time and energy to them. Even in the business world there is now considerable doubt as to the value of the MBA and although in management interviews candidates' possession of an MBA may get them on to the short list, I have been struck by how little attention is paid to it during the actual business of selection. Forty per cent of people with MBAs leave their company within a year of obtaining the MBA, in two cases out of three this is said to be because the employer failed to reward the possession of an MBA; this occurs especially in the public sector.[8] In fairness, however, one should add that many managers have said that it was a seminal intellectual event in their lives and felt that the effort was well worthwhile.

Explicit clinical back-up arrangements

Unless you are underemployed you cannot take on any significant clinical management role without giving up some clinical work. At first sight it may seem that this will not be necessary; but I and many other clinical managers have learnt by bitter experience that clinical management is not an add-on role. It must be an explicit part of your timetable. For this reason before accepting any clinical management post you will need to examine your clinical timetable and discuss with the chief executive or medical director how the necessary space is to be freed up in your timetable. This may require you dropping some sessions; colleagues may need to take up these sessions or it may even be necessary to appoint new clinical staff to take on the work. If either of the latter happen you must make absolutely certain, in writing, that those sessions will revert to you when you complete your term in clinical management.

"Re-entry" arrangements

It is very easy to get caught up in the business of clinical management to the neglect of your clinical practice and your continuing clinical education. You will, in addition, almost certainly have given up some clinical work to enable you to be a clinical manager. These factors can make it quite difficult to re-enter clinical practice smoothly at the end of your time in management, and unless the necessary arrangements have been made in advance, you may even be trapped into a situation where you may not wish to remain in clinical management long term but it becomes your predominant skill. I would suggest therefore, that at the outset of your appointment to a clinical management post you ensure that it is explicit and in writing that when you return to your clinical post you will have the same number of sessions to return to and that some arrangements will be made to allow whatever retraining is necessary. My Trust is both far-seeing and generous in that it allows senior clinical managers sabbatical leave of three months after three or more years in post and pays for attendance at courses, etc during that sabbatical leave. That seems to me to be a proper way of managing these things and ought to be the norm for all NHS trusts, though most will not be able to afford it.

2.5 How much will I be paid?

Some medical directors earn more than £100 000 a year when their clinical and managerial salaries and managerial perks are added together, but before you get too excited it must be pointed out that this is untypically high—although still chicken feed next to the million-dollar salaries of medical directors in the USA—and substantially more than most clinicians in management may expect.

Most clinical directors are paid the equivalent of one or two clinical sessions; medical directors perhaps five sessions or more.

2.6 Conclusion

You will have noted that I have assumed in this chapter that you will be moving into medical management and then, in due course, back to your original clinical role. It is probable that you will slip in and out of management over your career, but on current evidence fewer than 10% of clinical managers will stay in medical management as a long term major activity, and only a handful will give up their clinical work to become full-time managers, if only because most must have realised that to do so would lose them their "street credibility". Because of this tangential relationship with management it is critically important for clinicians, before they embark on this route, to view it as if they were piloting an untried aircraft. "Am I sufficiently trained for this flight?", "Is the vehicle in which I am flying airworthy?", "What will happen to me during the flight?", and "Have sufficient preparations been made for me to make a smooth landing?" The use of that simple analogy could spare you and your institution a lot of heartache.

References

1   Zeldin T. *An Intimate History of Mankind*. London: Minerva, 1995, pp 147–65.
2   Van Maurik J. *The Portable Leader*. London: McGraw Hill, 1997, p. 5.
3   Peters T. *Thriving on Chaos*. London: Macmillan, 1987.
4   Pendleton D, King J. Values and leadership. *BMJ* 2002;**325**:1352–5.
5   Micklethwait J, Wooldridge A. *The Witch Doctors*. London: Mandarin, 1997.
6   Peters T, Waterman R. *In Search of Excellence: Lessons from America's Best Run Companies*. New York: Harper & Row, 1982.
7   Bickerstaffe G. Ed. *Which MBA?* Economist Intelligence Unit, 13th Edn. London: Pearson, 2001.
8   Welch J. *People Management* 1997;**3**:12.

3: The medical manager's work

3.1 What do medical managers do?

This chapter concerns itself with what medical managers actually do and, to a lesser extent, what they ought to do. The latter is dealt with more fully in Section 4.9, "Professional and personal development". We noted at the outset that medical management includes a wide range of roles, including educational roles such as clinical tutor and postgraduate dean. The titles of those appointed to mainstream management positions in trusts range from "Lead Clinician", "Chief" or "Chair of the department", "Service Director", "Head of division", etc, but more than 80% are called "Clinical Director". The job of "Medical Director" is an explicitly different one.

The clinical director

Information on what clinical directors actually do is derived primarily from a British Association of Medical Managers (BAMM) survey published in 1997.[1] That survey found that most clinical directors *worked* 2·5 to five sessions at management tasks (the average being 3·12), but their average *contracted* time was 1·62 sessions (that is, one or two sessions). Therefore, most clinical directors can expect to work for twice as long as their contract predicts. Eighty-four per cent managed a budget and that budget ranged from £50 000 to £20 million. The most common was £2–3 million. Contentiously, though, this was usually not the whole budget for the clinical director's area of responsibility. In particular, it tended to exclude information technology, capital items, equipment replacement, nursing, recruitment, and theatre services. Having said that, of the 69% of clinical directors providing a list of principal items in their budget, the order of frequency of mentioning items was:

- hospital charges
- staff salaries
- pharmacy/drugs
- disposable/consumables
- equipment and its maintenance
- computers and IT consumables
- support services
- capital charges
- training and education.

It is an interesting aside in the document that although 66% of clinical directors were able to use savings generated in their budgets, 34% were not, which is hardly a stimulus to budgetary prudence.

When it comes to summarising the roles of clinical directors, one study has abbreviated them as:

- budget management
- business planning
- corporate decision making
- overall clinical and service direction
- quality assurance
- staff management

or more prosaically as:

- appoint clinical and support staff
- define and negotiate contracts
- purchase equipment
- quality issues and the handling of complaints
- staff disciplinary procedures
- strategic planning
- whole or partial responsibility for directorate budget.[2]

These jobs divide themselves into housekeeping tasks, such as personnel, budget details and purchasing, for which clinical directors should oversee the tasks where their clinical knowledge is important; and those that cannot be done as well by non-clinical managers, especially defining directorate strategy, using their clinical knowledge of the directorate. Clinical directors are particularly well placed to determine what actions within the directorate may be taken to exploit strengths and support weaknesses. It is also necessary for clinical directors to negotiate with purchasers to ensure realistic and achievable contracts are entered into, to decide which areas need quality improvement, and to lead that improvement. Lastly, clinical directors need to be able to sense when targets are not being met, despite what is said to them, and to act accordingly.

There are some areas which clinical directors are edged into, and you will need to take your own counsel as to whether they are proper tasks.

One such is the detail of *contracting*, which is a highly complex area. Although you need to understand the difference between different types of contract, such as "Block" and "Cost and Volume", and to understand the effect of these on the function of your directorate, fundamentally you should be supporting rather than leading the process.

Another difficult area is *marketing*. This popped on to the agenda in the wake of the market-style reforms of the NHS that came with "Working for Patients" and quickly began to appear as chapters in books on medical management (chapters almost never written by doctors). As the Thatcherite ethos of competition moderated, the push to market services reduced but will reappear with "Foundation Hospitals". Marketing as a concept means different things to different people, but to most of us it implies not simple provision of what is requested but actively selling a product. In this case the product is a skill, and actively selling means going beyond what is asked of you as a provider, and attempting to create a market. Apologists will say that marketing is, in fact, all about researching what the public wants and tailoring your product to their needs. That is not, I think, what the general public understands by marketing. We get into difficult areas here. Clinical teams with specialist skills may wish to attract patients and may even produce "advertising" material to underpin and communicate pride in their service. However, there is a narrow line between this and aggressive unit-against-unit marketing. What is important is that clinical directors are aware of the constructive features of this communications exercise in marketing and ensure that the facts that underpin the advertising are available when debates with purchasers take place. An exception perhaps is where a service needs more patients to function optimally and so clinical directors may need to actively go out to new purchasers and look for that work. In the current style of the NHS, though, these things should be part of sensible, cooperative negotiations about rationalisation and location of services, and not a "go get it", "winners and losers" kind of approach. But you may disagree with me about this.

Clinical directors do what they do largely for historic reasons; put crudely, doctors needed to do the dirty managerial jobs to bring them to their economic senses and to use them as agents to control their colleagues and thus the budget. We ought to have grown out of this now but many clinical directors feel used, undervalued, and not part of the core decision-making processes of their organisations. Too many are also involved in straightforward managerial chores that any manager could do (possibly better). The point has been made that we are an underdoctored country and cannot afford to lose so many top clinicians to management posts—doctors who should have their shoulders to the clinical wheel. Their time in management should therefore be used efficiently; this means an increased strategic role and allocating them adequate administrative, clerical, and managerial support. Unfortunately, in order to let doctors into the central part of the decision-making process many organisations will need to change their "closed-door" cultures.

How does real life match up to this?

Once, tired of counting sheep at night, I got up and wrote down the problems that were currently taxing me as a clinical director. The list went as follows (it is not prioritised).

- New Deal hours—still not working, need to employ phlebotomists and nurse practitioners. On what budget?
- Registrar training—still no consultant sessions dedicated to this. Needs more sessions. Needs more budget.
- Continuity of care.
- Nurse recruitment—need to fund yet another overseas trawl.
- Alcoholic Mr X—still need written evidence.
- Purchasers want higher percentage day-case surgery—need paper to indicate difficulties of this in our deprived catchment area.
- Insufficient beds—medical outliers as ever. No prospect of cross-subsidy.

- Radiology cross-charging—up again due to "research activity".
- Study leave—excessive and uncontrollable for academics, still no funding though for junior study leave.
- Complaint—MP still harassing us over a purely vexatious claim. Does not know the facts but expects action of some sort.
- Short-listing for consultant anaesthetist (again).
- MRSA (again).
- Stocking problem—too many different hip prostheses. Need to persuade consultants to use a smaller range.
- Waiting-list computer software—problems (again).
- List of audit projects for purchaser—needed this week but no reply about last year's yet. Need to persuade them to compare same projects from different providers.
- Finance director—still asking for £400k out of the budget!
- Prepare talk for management development seminar.
- Respond to Specialist Advisory Committee (SAC) document summarising their visit.

And those were just the directorate's problems and excluded Trust-wide issues.

It is said that good managers can deal with a maximum of five problems at a time. Ideally they should ask their personal assistants to type them onto a small card, which is kept handy in a suit pocket for ready reference. It is not like that. But perhaps therein lies the buzz of management and the real message should be not so much that there should be five problems, but that effective managers should be solving no more than five problems at any one time.

The medical director

"Medical Director" is a statutory post on the trust's board and is not the same as the old post of medical superintendent nor, it must be stressed, are medical directors the consultant's representative on a trust board. They are appointed by the chairperson and non-executive directors of the board with the chief executive's advice. Although not the representative of clinicians in the trust, it would be foolish to appoint someone who did not carry the approval of the consultant body.

Once appointed, medical directors are full and equivalent members of the board, they are directors of trusts and have a peer relationship with the chief executive and other board members, and share with them corporate responsibility for policy and decision making within the trust and the shaping of objectives. Medical directors are managerially responsible to the board and are not the chairperson's, nor the chief executive's, "medical poodle"—being less prisoners of the status quo than clinical directors.

Just as all executive members of the board have specific responsibilities, so too do medical directors. Their responsibilities are not statutorily defined and will vary from trust to trust. The wide range of those tasks was defined in a document produced by the Association of Trust Medical Directors in 1996, which enquired of more than 250 medical directors what their roles were.[3] The list produced is too onerous to be achieved by any one medical director; a better summary is the generic one produced by the Central Consultants and Specialists Committee in its document, *CCSC Guidance for Developing the Role of Medical Directors*. The CCSC identified the core tasks of the medical director, which in current parlance could be described as:

- providing professional medical advice to the trust board and its officers
- providing medical input to the development of strategy and strategic thinking
- communicating the trust perspective to clinicians
- supporting the work and development of clinical directors
- taking a key role in dealing with poorly performing colleagues
- overseeing the process of clinical risk and crisis management
- taking part in consultant appointment procedures and discretionary points and merit award systems
- overseeing clinical governance.

In all these tasks medical directors need to be more than just doctors. They need to develop new and different networks from those they had as doctors and to bring in ideas for clinicians from outside their normal milieu. These tasks will probably occupy at least five sessions a week. Whereas clinical directors are appointed by a range of mechanisms, from chief executive's whim to Buggin's turn, the process of appointing medical directors is much more defined and properly should be advertised and interviews held with representatives from the board present who will have taken soundings. Medical directors should be respected, or at least credible, as clinicians and therefore ought not to be full time in post. Neither should they concurrently be clinical directors so as to avoid clashes of priority or obligation. As with clinical directors, there is a risk that they will become bogged down in mundane issues that do not require clinical input. It is crucial that there is appropriate managerial and administrative support for them.

For medical directors, as for clinical directors, the trick is to escape from the jobs that are merely "housekeeping" and to try and concentrate on the tasks that support improvement and innovation, and to make these not just reactive but visionary, looking beyond the obvious next step.

3.2 Nurses and management

The two great professions of medicine are doctoring and nursing. Traditionally, they worked together in a comprehensible, synergistic way—doing different tasks but with doctors recognised as the dominant partners. Many of us have spent the majority of our professional lives in this environment in which it is accepted that the doctor is the clinical decision maker. However, the relationship between doctors and nurses has changed, and continues to do so, with no clear end in sight. The changes are important for medical managers for four reasons.

- Nurses form the greatest part of the hospital workforce.
- Their management by doctors is a contentious area.
- Healthcare may only be delivered effectively when doctors and nurses work together with clearly identified roles.
- The national and increasing shortage of nurses will force changes in the pattern of what they do.

So, without apology, there follows a brief history lesson on changes in nursing which have occurred over the past 30 years, because without that the present stresses and changes in nursing cannot be understood by medical managers. For the detail I am primarily indebted to Rivett's account of the history of the NHS.[4]

The development of nursing

Although the profession of nursing arose as much from a reaction against the drunken slatterns who supervised the filthy inmates of hospital wards before the end of the nineteenth century as it did from dedicated religious orders of earlier times, it is to the latter that we owe the concept of service that was formalised into a moral framework. To most people, nursing still represents a vocational ideal and, until recently, the attributes of the nurse were always considered to be those of "dedication, kindness, compassion, patience, trustworthiness, self-control, discretion, humility, perseverance, courtesy, the obedience of loyalty and respect".[5] Inherent in this position were not just huge status, but also low pay, subservience to doctors and even depersonalisation to an extent. Until recently ward sisters at St Thomas' were known by their ward and had no names of their own. This sounded fine when there were nice ward names and you could be called "Sister Alexandra" or "Sister Florence" but it depersonalised the sister and, anyway, it did not have quite the same ring when you were called "Sister X ray" or "Sister Gynae. Outpatients".

The status was stable from the time of Florence Nightingale until the 1960s, when both society and hospital practice began to change. Nursing came to be seen as a temporary job with high recruitment and high wastage, and hospitals' shortened stay and increased dependency significantly increased the pressures of working as a nurse. Until the 1960s education for nurses had been seen primarily as a practical activity to be undertaken at the bedside, apart from some theoretical knowledge passed on by medical staff. From the 1960s a desire for a more explicit education for nurses came to the fore and nursing education, for right or wrong reasons, became more and more to resemble the education of medical students; indeed, from now on it is likely that much nursing and medical student education at undergraduate level will be undertaken jointly.

Nursing was—and still is—predominantly a female profession. In the 1960s, women's rights and feminism were abroad. Education was seen as liberation and specifically in this case was identified as freedom from the shackles of primarily male doctors and from the passive role of selfless service and caring that reflected discredited domestic roles.

The propaganda for women was that this kind of activity was no longer to be seen as rewarding or appropriate. The development of nursing was led increasingly by educationalists and the theories that drove them mostly came from over the Atlantic. In May 1986 the proposals that were to become Project 2000 were lodged. Project 2000 was to transform the nature of student nursing so that students were no longer educated on the ward, no longer a pair of hands while being educated. The legacy of Florence Nightingale was at last defunct and, despite government anxiety about the cost and staffing implications of Project 2000, it was accepted; it was envisaged at the same moment that the hands-on work of patient care would in many ways be replaced by a new grade of support workers. Nursing, in a professional and educational sense, had changed but had to some extent gained a power to fashion its own direction, and what we have seen since then is experimental and theoretical attempts going in many different directions—some frustrating, most confusing watchers—and indeed many confusing nurses themselves.

The developments occurring in nursing have been fuelled by inescapable changes in health care, such as higher patient turnover, higher dependency, the need for discharge planning, the empowerment of patients, quality assessment exercises, and the disappearance of social workers from the wards. Unfortunately, the fact that many changes have been dressed up in educationalist, socialist or feminist political jargon has not helped. New concepts have involved "team nursing", the concept of "the named nurse". These fragmented the original cohesive concept of the ward, which doctors recognised as working so well. The concept of "the nursing process" was imported from the USA and required a formal and systematic review and documentation of patients' needs and a plan for dealing with them—"The Care Plan". Nurses developed paperwork of their own, running parallel to the doctor's clinical record, and doctors noticed that nurses spent more time writing or in huddles around Sister's desk than at patients' bedsides. Nursing had begun to run parallel to medicine.

The upheaval in nursing did, to the enormous benefit of health care, spawn nurses who were able to practise independently in a way that previously only midwives and district nurses had done: the nurse specialist, the nurse practitioner, nurse counsellors, independent midwives, etc. By this time the Royal College of Nursing was able to admit that not only was nursing separate from medicine in its day-to-day care of patients, but even accepted that nursing goals might differ from clinical goals. Many nurses found this empowering. Many found it deeply worrying, but whatever you believed, an unfortunate side-effect, as Rivett has noted, is that the political distance between doctors and nurses was widening at a time when they needed to be cohesive to resist outside threats to patient care.

Nursing and management

It was at the upper end of the nursing hierarchy that change was most profound, and for medical managers it is most important to understand and empathise with the ramifications of those changes.

Before the 1970s the shape of nursing hierarchy was absolutely clear. Matron was in charge, "her" ward sisters were responsible to her, and the ward nurses were responsible to sister. A neat, comprehensible, and functional family unit; but society has changed. Hospital is no longer the focus for a nurse's life. Turnover has increased, loyalty has wavered and this cosy family structure apparently is no longer appropriate. Additionally, there was a continuing problem of no real career spaces between ward sister and matron. The shortages of senior posts at this level made it difficult for nurses to influence the overall management of hospitals, and many nurses never achieved promotion beyond sister grade and the relatively inadequate salaries that this attracted.

The Salmon Report of 1966 inserted tiers of nursing administration above sister, the old concept of matron as a kind of "Mother Superior" figure disappeared, and the involvement of nurses in management as the only way to a higher salary was established. In management matters they had several heads' start over doctors, whose influence at this stage was still by committee. Nurses trained themselves in management but their management only ran to the management of nurses, they never really got a grip on the central power base of hospitals or of the NHS. The Griffiths Report of 1983, which brought in the concept of general management, is said to have regarded nurses as "doe-eyed and dangerous" and its reforms left nurses with no meaningful role. They have continued to exist in the shadows of non-clinical administrators and managers, and even though directors of nursing sit at the top table as full board members, their salaries are scandalously lower than those of their managerial peers around the table and their powers are very constrained.

When clinical management structures began to evolve in the wake of the Griffiths Report, the directorates that were set up often had one or more nurse managers. However, to this day it is unclear whether the intention was for nurse managers to manage nurses or to be managers who also happened to be nurses.

The commonsense arrangement which can apply in clinical directorates is a triumvirate of managers: a doctor manager; a nurse manager; and a non-clinical manager. However, the situation has now evolved to a point where, as best one can judge, many nurses who are managers are accepted as equivalent to any other manager but whose special skills happen to be in nursing just as another manager's might be in personnel or finance. In this arrangement the doctor medical manager is potentially often in a difficult position in relation to the nurses in the directorate. It may be that they are technically under his "command", yet they remain professionally accountable to matron's successor, the director of nursing, and in the midst of this is the nurse manager who is uncomfortably seated part way between the clinical director and the director of nursing. The nurse in that role may find her role potentially compromised by having to satisfy two separate agendas: the professional development of nurses and their responsibility to the patients as one-to-one carers; and at the same time satisfying a management agenda that may wish to look critically at nursing establishment, nursing practices, etc. This is the same dilemma as clinical directors can find themselves facing, and in fact, it should encourage both clinical directors and nurse managers to share their difficulties and their solutions. The position of nurses on the executive of trusts is no easier. A Royal College of Nursing study carried out in 1996 surveyed 340 nurse executive directors.[6] The report showed that these executive directors—trust board members— had a large range of job titles, 56 in total, yet interestingly less than a quarter were responsible for managing nursing services. The tendency was for them to manage low-budget areas without line management responsibilities. As alluded to above, their salaries are lower than those of other board members. Half those surveyed said they were the lowest paid board member—25% wanted to leave, 47% wanted to change their jobs within the next two years, and only 14% wanted to stay on until retirement.

In view of the size of the nursing workforce, its increasing level of education, both undergraduate and postgraduate, its commitment to change and to managerial training, it is depressing that nurses have not yet established a larger role in the machinery of the NHS. One can only hope that this will improve in the future. As far as individual medical managers are concerned, the starting point when establishing a relationship with nurses in management is to realise that they will probably be closest to them in terms of professional instincts and are natural allies. The medical manager must, however, bear in mind that all is not well in the world of nursing. To quote Ann Bradshaw:

> a split has formed between graduate nurses and vocational nurses who carry out practical tasks. Elitist nursing, intellectually unable to convince healthcare reformers of the need for advanced nursing practice, has alienated the vocational and practical majority of nurses ... UK nursing theory has displaced plain and simple caring, but not for a hard, technical science akin to medicine. Rather, social science dominates academic nursing knowledge and technique. Art and science have both been displaced and deconstructed, but is this breakdown beneficial for the care of patients? In the primary interest of patients, an informed, dispassionate and rational debate is needed in the public arena to consider the nature and purpose of nursing and nurse training.[5]

There are a lot of issues here that managers need to deal with; not just the dangers of gender politics but also the practical ones of a demoralised, underrewarded, underempowered group right at the heart of the organisation. Somehow, a career structure has to be found that incorporates the old loving habits of bedside nursing, meaningful incorporation in the wider management of the service, and a career development programme that does not depend at its upper end on the achievement of yet more classroom-based qualifications.

The NHS Plan with its stress on breaking down traditional boundaries between professional groups within the NHS may be the catalyst needed to allow nursing to escape its feminist, managerialist, politically correct bonds and refocus on real clinical issues. The development of the posts of "Nurse Consultant" and "Modern Matron" is a good omen for this.

3.3 Committees

Committees are the lifeblood of oligarchic management, but as any haematologist will tell you, too much blood is a bad thing, it slows the circulation and can lead to thrombosis. To you, as a manager, committees will sometimes seem to have a life of their own, a malevolent alien life force sucking the energies of the organisation. However, if they are managed well by the chairperson and participants, they can move the process of management ahead speedily and effectively, but if they are managed badly they are one of the most frustrating wastes of time that you are likely to experience. I am saddened by the waste of time, talent and money reflected in getting together the people who attend those meetings; meetings in which multidisciplinary, well-behaved worthies sit about exchanging platitudes, bemoaning the difficulties, pledging cooperative working after in-depth reappraisals—where sharp-nosed "chairs" call everyone by their Christian names and make a point of not leaving out the silent, dowdy individual from Community Health. And at the end of it there is frequently no conclusion, no plan of action that will be honoured, no righteous anger sent back up the line, no conspiratorial refusal to implement the unfunded and the unimplementable, no passionate plan to make happen what needs to happen, just a few well-rounded phrases in the minutes leading nowhere except to another committee meeting. It need not be like this!

You will, of course, have your own views about committees, but while the pressure sores of eight years on committees remain painful and unhealed, I hope I am allowed some observations.

Any committee

Make sure you have set aside time from your clinical or other work so that you arrive promptly and can stay until the end of meetings. Clinicians have a very bad reputation for arriving late in their white coats looking smug and leaving early as if to see patients, but probably because they are bored. Always, always read the paperwork before the meeting, and if it did not reach you at least 24 hours beforehand remonstrate at the meeting itself.

If there is an item on the agenda that is important to you, and for which you need support, try to talk to potential supporters and potential opponents before the meeting rather than expect to win them over during the meeting. Similarly, if the item is important sit where the chairperson can see you. If important decisions are made annotate your agenda papers with what was said and ensure that the minutes, when they subsequently emerge, reflect accurately what was agreed at the meeting.

If you are minded to set up a committee

Consider whether it is to achieve a defined purpose. If so, consider calling it a "working party", give it a written remit and a timetable. If a formal remit cannot be framed then it is almost a corollary that the committee will be without influence.

An unsatisfactory reason for setting up a committee is merely to allow colleagues to meet for a chat about mutually interesting issues. Even less acceptable are meetings to appease complaints about exclusion from the decision-making process by establishing a toothless talking shop.

If the committee is for the purpose of conducting necessary routine business (the usual reasons for having a committee)

It is important to know to whom the committee reports, whether it has an executive function, and who sets the agenda. If you can not answer these questions then perhaps the committee should not exist, and you should consider whether some other less formal grouping will fulfil the task that you have in mind.

If you have been made chairperson of a committee

If the committee meets regularly, try to arrange for it to meet at intervals which may be calculated monthly or quarterly, and for meetings to be held at the same time and day of the week.

A meeting with constantly changing times may seem a good idea in that no small group of members are particularly put out by having to change their timetables, but it invariably leads to confusion and is usually deemed unsatisfactory and scrapped.

When considering timing, clinicians tend to find a five o'clock meeting or later the most convenient if it is to be a one- or two-hour meeting, but major meetings that will last at least three hours should be timetabled as a half day. Some like breakfast meetings, "power breakfasts", though personally I think they are a sin for they encapsulate all the failures of the machismo management culture, namely:

- failure to plan working timetables effectively
- I can get up earlier than you!
- failure to respect the private lives of contributors.

They are also gastronomically a disaster.

It has been noted that the length of committee meetings is proportional to the weight of the chairperson. Thinner chairs become hypoglycaemic and restive more quickly. Chairs (chairpersons has dropped out of common usage you may be pleased to note) bear the responsibility for making committees work smoothly and productively; so decide in advance the length of meetings, the important issues that must be decided upon and those that may be allowed to drift for a while. If important but contentious decisions are to be made try to talk with the key players beforehand. Try to make sure that the quiet members get as much chance to have their say as the pushy ones. Lastly, train your antennae to sense the ploys people use to manipulate meetings.

The conduct of committees

Remember that committees subserve several different functions:

- information transmission
- commenting on and potentially altering proposed decisions
- a truly open-ended debate on an issue with the purpose of formulating policy.

When managing the agenda of a meeting it is important that you are clear into which category each item will fall. Agendas may usefully be divided into items "for information", "for decision", or "for discussion". Where there is clear division firm "chairship" is needed to ensure the players keep to it. There is a lot of Brownian movement in committees, grumbling and rumbling, to-ing and fro-ing, and this tends to amplify itself so that all committees have an inbuilt tendency to chaos. The more democratic and openly run they are the worse the risk. The danger in this is that the committee may fail to make decisions and those decisions are then merely made on another day by a smaller group. There is a theoretical ideal composition for a committee, the character of whose different members so complement one another that the committee works perfectly. Psychologists love to appraise and analyse top teams (ideally for a fee) to see that there is the right mix of initiators, finishers, lateral thinkers, healers, etc. In the real world, of course, one does not have the luxury of picking the perfect mix, which anyway may not be as important as theorists assert; indeed, one of the most functionally effective committees I have ever been on was assessed by professional psychologists to be, in theory, totally dysfunctional.

Ploys

You should be aware of a number of ploys that (other) people use in committees to get their own way.

- *Bludgeoning.* This is probably the simplest manoeuvre, it simply involves monopolising the conversation or the agenda until you get your own way, or refusing to support other people until they support you. This tends to be a surgeon's ploy; surgeons lust after action (often for its own sake), whereas physicians, happy in the cosy inglenooks of the intellect, prefer a quiet debate.
- *Any Other Business.* The item is slipped in at the end of the meeting under "Any Other Business" when the members are tired and some have left. Items for "Any Other Business" should therefore be declared at the beginning of the meeting.
- *Filibustering.* Sometimes you may think this is deliberate when it's simply unstructured locquaciousness, which

reminds me of John Major's comments about Neil Kinnock "Since he did not know what it was he was trying to say he had no way of knowing when he had finished!"

- *The Tabled Paper.* This is where the paper presenting your argument is slipped onto the table during the meeting and other members of the committee have neither the time to read the paper nor the opportunity to check the facts. Tabled papers should not be allowed.
- *Awaiting the absence of opponents.*
- *The Trojan Horse Manoeuvre.* This involves embedding the subject of your choice into some other non-contentious issue, either in the agenda papers or in the debate.
- *The Go-between Manoeuvre.* This is a variant of the Trojan Horse manoeuvre and involves using a biddable and acceptable messenger to achieve your ends rather than putting it up yourself when people may be sensitised to you or your message.
- *Misrepresentation* of what the committee actually decided. Although this sounds like straightforward dishonesty it is, I suspect, more often simply that you hear what you wish to hear. Always check the minutes of the last meeting.

Are committees effective?

It would be nice to think that they are, and it is a fact of life to discover that often they are not, but that should not dismay you. The alternatives after all are likely to be less palatable stop-off points on the continuum between dictatorship and mob rule. Committees are after all just part of the management process in which team members come together, and teams do not necessarily work well together but you can assist the process by ensuring that committees are small enough to function efficiently yet not so small as to exclude key players. You can get almost any committee to work if you have properly prepared papers sent out in good time, a competent chairperson adequately briefed, and lastly, participants who accept the discipline needed to get through the business in time and make decisions.

A word about "Brainstorming" and "away days". Particularly with the former there is sometimes a naive assumption that these free-for-all sessions, uncluttered by pagers and preconceptions will throw up solutions not previously thought of—they do not, but they do run the particular risk of falling under the spell of the ardent, articulate, well-prepared participant; so make sure that is you!

3.4 Time management

Controlling stress in the job

Taking on a management role while continuing as a clinician is a recipe for stress. This needs to be realised at the outset and steps taken to control it. Caplan's study of stress in GPs, hospital consultants, and hospital managers showed depression in 27%, 19%, and 6%, respectively,[7] although depression need not of course be just a response to stress. Another study, by contrast, has shown that one in three NHS managers are suffering from stress, a figure approximately similar to doctors and nurses.[8,9] What is not yet known is what surplus stress or depression levels, if any, are experienced by clinicians who are also managers. Are natural copers selected for the job or do the conflicts and the workload inherent in the double job lead to stress symptoms? Or, does having your hand on the reins protect from stress. From personal observations I have no doubt that "burn-out" can occur in clinician managers because of the insoluble frustrations of the job, just as it can in oncologists. Whether the stresses of clinical and management work done in parallel are synergistic needs to be explored. A study performed for the Association of Surgeons of Great Britain and Ireland[10] explored conflicts between administrative, clinical, and personal life. There was a response from 305 of 975 Fellows. Seventy per cent described a conflict between administrative work and personal life during the previous three weeks, with 78% being resolved in favour of the administrative demand. Seventy-one per cent also reported conflicts between clinical and administrative work during the previous three weeks, with 49% being resolved in favour of the administrative demands. Worryingly 68% believed their work with patients had suffered at least once during the previous month because of stress. That study was conducted in 1994 and the conflicts and stresses are certainly worse now.

What is clear is that the management of time is central to the management of stress, and that a little thought invested in planning time management at the outset of your appointment will pay dividends later. Management of the flow of information is also critical, though perhaps less easy to assess than problems with time management.

Time management

It is not natural for people to admit that they waste a good deal of their time at work, particularly when they see themselves as overworked, but bear in mind the Bareto 80/20 principle. Bareto was a nineteenth-century economist who noted that, for example, 20% of the workforce does 80% of the work, 20% of a document contains 80% of the useful information and so on. It must be assumed that your work potentially displays the same split and in arranging to manage time you want to get rid of as much of the 80% non-productive work as is possible. If you do not manage this you may find yourself with an uncontrolled workload, punishing your family or yourself to the point when new and even more damaging stresses are introduced into your life. To cope with all this you need some strategies and the strength of purpose to observe them.

Firstly, you need a *personal job plan*, a personal declaration of intent about how you plan to lead your life as a manager. This need not be public, it can be in your head, although if it is shared with your domestic partner it will be less easy to deny later that these were your objectives. For example:

> I am the clinical director for acute medical directorates. In addition to this I will take an interest in things to do with emergency medicine, primary care and elderly care. I am not personally interested in computing, junior doctors hours or registrar training programmes, so I will avoid or delegate these. I will have breakfast with my children every day and will accept evening obligations on only two days a week. I will arrange events to allow me to visit the gym on Tuesdays and Thursdays at 6.00 pm, etc.

A bit short but the right flavour. Having done that, now some specific tactics.

Tactic one—a hard relook at the timetable

Have you yet scheduled one or more half days when you are in your office? You need to do that and to ensure that your secretary (now that you are a manager you will be calling him or her a PA!) knows that this is the only time to arrange for people to see you. Have you scheduled a regular team meeting and/or a walkabout session? All these should count as managerial "fixed sessions" in addition to any predictable committee work.

Tactic two—dealing with the mail

There are many ways to solve this problem; for example get your PA to sort the mail into four separate heaps. Firstly, the clinical mail; secondly, managerial material needing letters; thirdly, managerial documents needing reading; and, fourthly (usually the largest pile) material that can be thrown into the bin, for example invitations to seminars, the third blurred photocopy of the latest executive circular, advertising material, etc. Additionally you will need a carefully garnered pile of papers relating to impending committees. These should be clearly labelled, because everything nowadays is printed in Times New Roman typeface on "Word" and looks identical. Ideally, it should be presented in a separate file containing the agenda, minutes of the last meeting, etc.

Try not to leave in the evening before you have dealt with the mail and dictated on it where necessary. Just dumping it all into your briefcase to be dealt with at home is not the correct solution. Although you should try not to handle any piece of mail more than once, a "pending file" is useful. Things you think are probably unimportant but you are not entirely sure can be put in the file. When you check the file in three months' time you will find most of it can go straight into the bin.

Treat email in the same way as letters. If you set about reading your emails on screen you will be quickly bogged down in trivia and irrelevance, quite apart from suffering stress generated by the slovenly abuse of language that typifies them. If your system allows it, exclude junk emails by setting your mail box to accept only mail addressed to you personally.

Tactic three—avoid interruptions

It is difficult to balance accessibility with the need to work effectively. Your clinical colleagues are the most difficult in this. Not only will they expect you to be able to fix things for them but they also want to tell you about it, at length—now!

Very few people understand the stresses under which you work and few of them respect your time. Therefore leave your bleep or mobile phone with someone outside when you are going into a meeting, have all the calls to your office passed through your secretary, and lastly, remain standing and close to the door when people "drop by" to see you without an appointment. These manoeuvres can, of course, be carried to extremes and it is irritating when telephoning others to be told that they are "in a meeting". The retort "what meeting is that?" or "is it a real meeting?" may elucidate whether your target is simply chatting to a colleague and can be disturbed. Remember, however, to treat others as you would wish them to treat you and that however urgently you feel you need to talk to the chief executive or the director of finance, they are as likely to be as frustrated by unstructured calls on their time as you are.

Tactic four—avoid futile meetings

As a clinical or medical director you will be asked to many meetings simply from courtesy or because the arrangers wish to influence you. If the meeting is not part of your mainstream obligations or will not contribute to your personal objectives, do not accept. If you are in doubt as to whether this is the right course it is sometimes acceptable to ask if you could receive the minutes and agendas and come only if there are relevant items. You will have to learn to live with the anxiety that meetings you do not attend may decide something with which you do not agree.

Inherent in all this is the ability to say "No". New consultants and new medical managers tend to be flattered to be asked to do things and may not have a clear view of what saying "Yes" will entail. So, if asked, *always* find out what saying "Yes" lets you in for and then make a careful judgment in your own time rather than in the corridor. Saying "No" sounds selfish but it is not always so, it may be simply sensible.

Tactic five—delegate

This does not mean ducking your responsibilities; it is a positive act that ensures that other team members have their skills used properly. Delegation may also be used as a good vehicle with which to "bring on" clinicians who have no current management responsibilities. Even the smallest task exposes them to the *realpolitik* of making the system work. It is sensible though, when delegating in this way, to outline the task, though not necessarily the process, and to give a timetable in writing. Remember not to delegate work which should simply be eliminated.

There is a useful management aphorism about prioritisation: "Do it, delegate it, or discard it".

Tactic six—manage the flow of information

As doctors we have well-structured ways for handling information: we read a selected, small group of journals; and we know how we can retrieve that information via computer searches or by way of our personal filing system. We have books whose authors largely agree on how best to deal with any particular clinical problem. We go to meetings where the advice we receive is largely consensual and probably has some scientific validity. It then comes as a rude shock to the new manager to be quickly buried by an avalanche of unstructured information.

At first it is impossible to determine what is necessary, what is useful, what might be useful in the future, and indeed, to determine which of all this stuff is true, what is a try on, what is propaganda, and where is the kernel of this overripe information fruit that reports a policy which is real and will be acted upon. The information is presented untidily—heaps of verbose, expensively printed reports vie for your attention with binders full of undigested data, beguilingly glossy free magazines, emails, faxes, and photocopies slipped under the door by the invisible bumph fairy. The fruit of the information tree has an exceptionally low nutritional value even for a manager hungry to find out what it is that keeps this new world spinning. It is difficult to know what to file, what to open, what to read even, so the rookie manager needs quickly to learn the skills of skim reading, prioritisation and, most importantly, of throwing paper away. Be very wary of just putting things to one side or of filing them unread, for that only encourages an accusatory and depressing burden of information that will never be assimilable. A survey by Reuters found that half of 1300 managers questioned were suffering from a degree of information overload which, far from making their tasks easier as was intended, was actually leading to less ability to make a decision and to more stress.[11] The information overload does this simply because we are not able to assimilate the torrent of information and yet we feel we ought to, for within the unassimilated information might be the nugget that negates what we are about to decide. The urgency culture of mobile phones and emails implies that everything is genuinely important and can make the whole thing even more stressful. As this is a pandemic disease which society currently shows no desire to alleviate there is little individuals can do, but there is a lot to be said for *not* having a mobile phone, *not* having email, and leaving the answerphone switched off most of the time! Managerial matters are rarely that urgent and often benefit from maturing in an in-tray for a while or waiting to be aired at the next scheduled committee meeting.

Tactic seven—do all of this in the right environment

A good PA or secretary, an effective filing system, and a clear desk are essentials. Two to three comfortable chairs around a low table where you can have discussions are very helpful. You might even explore the Feng Shui approach. Feng Shui is the ancient Chinese art of correct placement; if things in your environment are placed appropriately your life will be happier, easier, and more successful. However, given the limitations of NHS space and budgets, your options for amending your environment with mirrors, large plants and wind chimes are likely to be seriously curtailed, so you may have to live with your chi running incorrectly through your space. The best you can do is avoid the omnipresent pressures of mounds of unresolved paperwork surrounding you on every flat surface. An empty desk is indeed a happy desk. I expect someone has said "Show me a cluttered office and I will show you a cluttered mind"—I hope not!

3.5 Managing a budget

I did not relish writing this section of the book. I am no exception in this; it is the management area that clinicians seem to like least. So I shared the problem with my undergraduate son when he was home for the weekend—"Managing a budget ... what's the problem? You get given an amount of money and you just have to make it last." Ah! If only it were that simple, but therein lies the answer to the clinician's difficulty.

Problems about budget holding

Undergraduates, apart from a need to keep their food intake above starvation level, and to buy the occasional round of drinks, are masters of all the elements of their budgets. Not so clinicians in management. They are probably aware that the evolving NHS created the concept of clinicians in management almost solely as an attempt to control clinical budgets; they may agree with the concept; they may understand intellectually and emotionally that money is real and budgets are finite, but they personally spend only a tiny part of the budget and most of the expenditure within their directorate is historically based, inescapable, or driven by factors outside their control. Clinical managers' scepticism about the virtues of budget holding will be further fuelled by the fact that they are unlikely to have encountered a part of the NHS in which poor budgetary performance has led to closure or firings. In contrast, they will be familiar with the time-honoured response of overspending budget holders being rewarded with an increase in budget, whereas underspenders are penalised by a reduction in next year's allocation. None of this is really a recipe for enthusiastic budget holding by clinicians. In addition, clinical managers may find the paperwork daunting unless it is properly presented and they have been educated to understand it. So, what should clinical managers understand?

- The types of budgets that exist in an NHS unit.
- How data is commonly presented to the budget-holding medical manager.
- How the budget is set.
- The sort of options that clinical directors have to control budgets and expenditure.

Types of budget

It is important to identify the two types of accounting activity that trusts and other NHS organisations undertake.

- *Financial accounting*—sometimes called "stewardship accounting". This is the accounting to the people who provide the money to show that it has been properly used. Such accounting is usually annual and historical, and will include items of income and expenditure, reviews of assets, use of capital, and so on. It is outside the scope of this chapter.
- *Management accounting*—this is the kind of accounting that medical managers will deal with and they should not be sceptical about the need for it. It is simply a management tool that involves the setting of budgets and the production of regular, useful accounts, usually on a monthly basis, that look back at expenditure and look forward to determine whether expenditure will match income. They seem natural now, but in 1978 the Royal Commission on the NHS noted an almost complete absence of them. The Thatcher government's "Working for Patients" in 1989, whatever its other failings, did at least help to establish prudent accountancy practice as a mainstream feature of NHS management. Management accounting should underpin the running of any business because, quite simply, it helps managers to balance income with expenditure and may help them to explore areas which need attention. Lastly, of course, it provides the data which allows them to write a credible business plan.

There is another sort of accounting "cost accounting"; this is a specialised discipline allowing accurate costing of products in the commercial sector. It is not generally used within the NHS.

As a clinical director you discover that there are two parts to the management accounting in relation to your service. One is the *central budget* which describes the core function of the organisation, including obvious things such as facilities, catering, rates, and electricity, and the less obvious items like reserves and capital charges. The other is your *directorate budget*, which concerns expenditure by your team in your directorate. When assessing costs, these two budgets must be reconciled.

The central budget is always larger than clinical directors think it ought to be, but defining it is a complex area left to the finance department. If, however, you are involved in price setting for contracts you will need to know the details of those central costs. You are, of course, allowed to be critical if they seem to be profligate.

Directorate budgets

Managing your own directorate budget will require you to slot into a budget cycle of *setting*, *reporting*, and *reviewing*, and then the familiar biological feedback cycle that also applies to audit, whereby the reviewing informs the next cycle of *setting* and so on.

Budget setting

This is done by the chief executive and/or the director of finance, but must involve you, your business manager, and finance manager, otherwise we fall into the old NHS trap of divorcing budget planning from operational management. Traditional budget setting occurs in advance of the financial year and is supposed to be concluded by March, although it may be difficult to achieve this if there are delays in concluding contracts, getting allocations and so on.

The budget as set is usually historical with extra cash allocated for medical advances, inflation, etc, together with additional contractual work. From this is subtracted any efficiency savings expected of you, or any fraction of an overall income loss that the trust is experiencing which is to be passed on to your directorate. Last year's overspend or underspend may also be reflected in this year's budget. All of that is the "top down" element.

The "bottom up" part of the process is what your clinical directorate brings to the debate. This is rarely part of the negotiation about the budget to be set, but is more often part of the process of looking to see how genuine cost pressures that your directorate may experience can be met from within your budget. Examples of such cost pressures might include the implementation of the European working time directive, or the separation of male wards from female wards. Also to be taken into account are initiatives arising from your own directorate business plan which you will want to put into your calculations. Remember when doing that that satisfying demands for information, for extra teaching, for audit, for quality improvements ought normally to have a price tag attached: "Yes, we'll happily do that but it will cost £xx in the next financial year". These figures also need to go into the brew. There is an element of negotiation between you and the director of finance in all this, but the finance director's room for manoeuvre will probably be very limited and your increased costs are unlikely to be reflected in extra income for the trust. At the end of this process you would, in traditional terms, be set a fixed budget, or possibly a partly flexible budget; the flexible element reflects unpredictable workloads beyond your control but only if this extra activity will be funded from elsewhere.

You will also at this point need to be clear what the plans are for the management of over- or underspends during the coming year, in particular whether you have an option to use *revenue* underspends on *capital* equipment and, lastly, what level of expenditure you are personally authorised to commit. The rules relating to the clinical director's power personally to approve expenditure differ from one organisation to another, but each will have "standing financial instructions" which you ought to read (very boring but very important!), especially in relation to the upper limits of spending which the clinical director is allowed.

The reforms since 1998 have made the budget-setting process more difficult. Expenditure control will remain as important as ever, but the "abolition" of the internal market made the ability to manage income potentially more difficult because income is more fixed than it was in the days of the "internal market" and less likely to be responsive to workload.

When the budget is finally set you *must* be clear what elements of the budget can be controlled and what can realistically be achieved. This is where your clinical knowledge is crucial and where everybody must be clear about what is controllable and what is not. The finance director and the chief executive also need to be clear about this. It does not do the organisation a favour to start the year with unreasonable or overoptimistic budgetary expectations, yet one sees it over and over again, leading to crises of cancellation and media interest each winter, usually echoed by government ministers blaming the service for inept management.

Cost improvement programmes

"Cost improvement" means "cost reduction", you cannot *improve* on a cost but *improvement* sounds good so it is there to blunt the sting. So abjectly submissive to these "weasel words"[12] have we become that I missed this one until none other than our director of finance pointed out how misleading the term is. Unfortunately, we are stuck with it.

If big chunks are to be taken out of the budget, either for an explicit cost improvement programme or because of a previous unresolved overspend, the mechanics of those savings should be explicit and agreed at the outset and communicated to all the team. There is nothing more depressing and unachievable for a clinical director than to be told part way through the year that the expected out-turn needs to be reduced by a large amount.

Specific cost improvement programmes must be accurately costed, their progress monitored and, in general, they should be achieved without a reduction in workload. Even if cost pressures are discounted, it becomes increasingly difficult year on year to achieve significant cost improvements once the obvious targets such as overstaffing, length of stay and day surgery rates have been addressed. Simply *not* doing things is the next option. For example, limiting the number of investigations or procedures for a disease or simplifying drug therapy. If this is to be done without reducing the quantity of care provided, it can only be informed by properly researched evidence-based medicine (EBM) protocols. There is of course a snag in this that for every cost-saving EBM protocol, there may be an equal number of cost-increasing protocols. The merging of clinical departments between hospitals is another option, but this rarely produces the large savings needed, even though such savings will usually have been adduced as the reason for a merger.

Budget reporting

The budget, once set, will need to be reported on monthly. If you, the clinical director, are going to be able to respond usefully to those reports, they will need to be:

- accurate
- timely
- understandable
- relevant
- consistent
- agreed.

There is no virtue in the report containing "fixed costs", such as rent and rates, and capital charges, because the clinical director cannot influence these. The actual report will need to show so-called "semi-fixed" costs, such as:

- nursing salaries
- consultant salaries
- administrative and clerical salaries

and "variable" costs such as:

- theatre charges
- cross-charges for meals and portering
- drugs
- pathology tests
- theatre disposables.

It will need clearly to identify agency and locum staff costs as these tend to be a source of nasty surprises.

The lines are subdivided into columns: the annual budget, sometimes called the plan; this month's budget; this month's actual spend; variance from the plan; and some sort of full-year projection with the variance to show how your budget is likely to end the year. Be familiar with the notations used, especially where it signifies an overspend. Figures in brackets may signify a gain or underspend, as they do in Figure 3.1, but in other organisations they may signify the opposite! To make managerial sense of these figures, you will also need to see some basic activity and staffing data, such as finished consultant episodes, admissions and waiting lists, again presented as predicted and actual figures. Lastly, it is helpful to know what your staff levels are in relation to establishment. It is sometimes possible to include all this data for a directorate on a single sheet of paper.

The trust as a whole will have similar but larger sheets covering all of its business, divided up by its separate component services.

You can try to use all this information to yield a price per procedure, or a cost per case. In theory this will allow you comparison between your patients and those of other services or directorates, or even other hospitals, but the variability in case mix, the crudeness of cost allocations and the primitiveness of NHS information technology, makes the figures largely meaningless. The drive to produce these figures

GUY'S AND St. THOMAS' NHS HOSPITAL TRUST 1998/99
FINANCIAL PERFORMANCE REPORT FOR THE PERIOD: APRIL TO JULY
VASCULAR SURGERY
99 S-03-831

WTE BUDGET	WTE ACTUAL	JULY BUDGET £	JULY SPEND £	JULY VARIANCE £	Code	Description	ANNUAL BUDGET £	TO DATE BUDGET £	TO DATE SPEND £	VARIANCE TO DATE £
						MEDICAL STAFF				
1·36	1·36	9065	8583	(482)	MC210	CONSULTANT	108769	36234	34402	(1832)
		3830	3552	(278)	MC21M	CONSULTANT MEDICAL SCHOOL	45963	15321	14984	(337)
		0	1452	1452	MN410	SENIOR REGISTRAR	0	0	16851	16851
2·00	1·00	8257	0	(8257)	MN250	SPEC REGISTRAR	99096	33000	12222	(20778)
		0	916	916	MN25M	SPR REGISTRAR	0	0	2748	2748
1·00	1·00	3316	11969	8653	MN210	SENIOR HOUSE OFFICER	39811	13254	11969	(1285)
3·00	3·00	6824	6463	(361)	MN110	HOUSE OFFICER	81890	27250	26064	(1186)
		0	13924	13924	MN25L	SPR REGISTRAR LOCUM	0	0	13924	13924
0·66	1·00	2156	0	(2156)	MN31L	REGISTRAR LOCUM	25891	8619	0	(8619)
		888	0	(888)	ZADH0	ADDITIONAL DUTY HOURS	10652	3551	931	(2621)
8·02	7·36	34336	46859	12523		TOTAL MEDICAL STAFF	412072	137229	134095	(3134)
						NURSING STAFF				
1·00	1·00	2131	2127	(4)	NX010	SNR NURSE PRACTITIONER	25568	8523	8509	(14)
1·00	1·00	2131	2127	(4)		TOTAL NURSING STAFF	25568	8523	8509	(14)
						ADMIN & CLERICAL				
1·00	1·00	1733	1706	(27)	CR31S	MEDICAL SECRETARY 4	20789	6930	6823	(107)
2·00		2941	(1704)	(4645)	C000M	ADMIN & CLERICAL MEDICAL SCH	35298	11766	13787	2021
		545	(1694)	(2239)	C000A	ADMIN & CLERICAL STAFF AGENCY	6550	2183	9327	7144
3·00	1·00	5219	(1692)	(6911)		TOTAL ADMIN & CLERICAL	62637	20879	29937	9058

WTE BUDGET	WTE ACTUAL	JULY BUDGET £	JULY SPEND £	JULY VARIANCE £			ANNUAL BUDGET £	TO DATE BUDGET £	TO DATE SPEND £	VARIANCE TO DATE £
						NON PAY				
		0	0	0	2B000	STAFF UNIFORMS	10	3	0	(3)
		6656	5355	(1301)	2D00E	Drugs Expend Cross Charge	79880	26627	28128	1501
		6914	5524	(1390)	2DHE1	Blood Products Exp Cross Charge	82967	27656	24380	(3276)
		12	0	(12)	2F000	MEDICAL & SURGICAL EQUIPMENT	150	50	0	(50)
		5590	0	(5590)	2G000	PATIENTS APPLIANCES	67080	22360	9235	(13125)
		0	2016	2016	2GSA0	surgical appliances	0	0	5191	5191
		7	0	(7)	2P000	ELECTRICAL APPLIANCES	90	30	0	(30)
		6	0	(6)	2W000	RESUS PRINTING & STATIONERY	73	24	12	(12)
		28	0	(28)	2WA00	COMPUTER HARDWARE	346	115	1463	1348
		186	0	(186)	2WH00	STATIONERY	2231	744	17	(727)
		99	0	(99)	3DA00	ADVERTISING COSTS	1183	395	0	(395)
		20	0	(20)	3DE01	TRAINING & ED COURSE FEES	230	77	250	173
		0	(403)	(403)	3DR00	REMOVAL EXPENSES	0	0	0	0
		152	0	(152)	3DT00	TRAVEL & SUBSISTENCE	1834	611	385	(226)
		7	0	(7)	3DT01	EXCESS TRAVEL EXPENSES	90	30	22	(8)
		89	515	426	3X00M	MED PHOTO-MED SCH RECHARGE	1072	357	715	358
		2	0	(2)	3X00P	PHOTOCOPYING - MED SCH RECHARGE	31	10	0	(10)
		17	0	(17)	3XM9M	MED/SCH ULTRASONIC ANGIOLOGY	204	68	0	(68)
		743	980	237	9AM80	PATIENTS TRANSPORT RECHARGE	8909	2970	3094	124
		2	0	(2)	9B000	MINI CAB/TAXI RECHARGES	24	8	0	(8)
		0	350	350	9BEDS	USE OF BEDS CROSS CHARGE	0	0	490	490
		56	0	(56)	9CC01	TELEPHONE RECHARGES	668	223	566	343
		21327	18406	(2921)	9EITU	ITU Recharges inwards	255928	85309	36826	(48483)
		679	281	(398)	9ENUC	EXP NUCLEAR MEDICINE RECHARGES	8141	2714	1123	(1591)

Figure 3.1

Code	Description							
9EPCH	EXP CHEM PATH TESTS	3245	4242	997	38957	12985	13853	868
9EPHA	EXP HAEMATOLOGY TESTS	3662	4826	1164	43940	14647	16723	2076
9EPHI	EXP HISTOPATHOLOGY TESTS	9717	16494	6777	116603	38868	50791	11923
9EPIM	EXP IMMUNOLOGY TESTS	186	560	374	2236	745	1506	761
9EPMI	EXP MICROBIOLOGY TESTS	3916	4108	192	46994	15665	15546	(119)
9EPVI	EXP VIROLOGY TESTS	262	600	338	3154	1051	1716	665
9ERAD	EXP RADIOLOGY INTERNAL RECHARG	28120	27664	(456)	337441	112480	115765	3285
9HOSP	CATERING HOSPITALITY RECHARGE	0	0	0	0	0	10	10
9PC00	IT TRAINING RECHARGES	10	0	(10)	120	40	0	(40)
9PC04	IT INSTALLATIONS/LICENCES RECH	0	0	0	0	0	100	100
9PH00	PHOTOCOPYING RECHARGE	0	0	0	0	0	5	5
9****	TOTAL INTERNAL RECHARGES	71925	78511	6586	863115	287705	258114	(29591)
	TOTAL NON PAY SPEND	91710	91517	(193)	1100586	366862	327912	(38950)
	TOTAL THIS REPORT	133396	138812	5416	1600863	533493	500453	(33040)
		12-02		9-36				

Figure 3.1 An example of a financial performance report. This is a monthly report for the clinical director of surgery and concerns the vascular surgical unit. The costs of theatre time, outpatients, and the use of the team's own beds are not included in this budget. The clinical director will see them on the report for the whole directorate.

was once an inherent need of the internal market and is still pursued for its own sake. Sadly, though, the NHS has never realised that information is not a free good, nor to my knowledge has there ever been a cost–benefit analysis of whether *detailed* knowledge of cost can be shown to alter the total cost of health care or to improve it within the NHS. In the USA and in the UK private sectors, where activity is largely funded on a cost-per-case basis, such costing activities are inescapable. Costing as an obsession, however, is here to stay and the case mix issue is being addressed; thus you may need to be familiar with the concept of diagnosis-related groups (DRGs). There are several hundred of these and, in theory, each can be separately costed, but they are crude. In the UK the tendency has been to use healthcare resource groups (HRGs), which are more sophisticated as they combine diagnosis, secondary diagnoses, and procedures. It may be possible to make them more accurate by adding severity scores. Eventually, perhaps, meaningful costings and maybe even outcome analyses will be available.

It is not your job as medical manager to construct these equations, but you do need to try to ensure that these complicated financial activities do not drift too far away from clinical reality. As far as your own budget sheet is concerned the structure and the figures need to be devised between your business manager and the finance directorate. You need to know not only the director of finance in your organisation but also the person responsible for monitoring and constructing your budget. In big hospitals with big finance departments this may be difficult but it is important for there to be an identifiable individual. Some would say that that person should be *managerially* accountable to you while *professionally* accountable to the director of finance. I am not convinced that accountability to you the clinical director is crucial, but it is important that a named person is responsible for the accuracy of your budget sheets.

Reviewing and controlling expenditure in a clinical directorate

So here you are at your monthly review meeting, cup of coffee in hand, budget statement in front of you, and your team eager to discuss what is needed.

An example of the sort of budget statement which you might have is shown in Figure 3.1 above.

It is "Month 4" (that is finance speak for July) and things are going well. There are some "year to date expenditures" which are less than planned. Can you spend the surplus? Probably not! Look very closely to see why this unusual state of affairs has obtained. There is a small overall underspend on medical staff but a big overspend on medical staff this month which you need to sort out because if it continues through the year it may wreck your budget. Staff underspends due to unfilled vacancies are OK, unless the staff agency bill simply has not been paid yet. Lower than expected use of consumables is OK, but only if it accurately reflects what has already been bought or committed which is very unusual. Non-pay expenditure is always difficult to track accurately because you need to measure expenditure commitments as well as actual expenditure. It is quite common for things to look good mid-year, only to slip as the year goes on. In the example shown here you can see that the ITU cross-charging budget is underspent, or is it? Again, you will need to know if this truly represents a change in practice leading to less demand for ITU beds or is it just the vagaries of the billing process or is it a temporarily low throughput. Also note on this budget sheet how financially trivial are many of the lines (where you might be tempted to act) and that there are big sums in some lines, such as blood products and radiology, where changed clinical practice might produce real savings if you need them.

In the more common scenario, either things are looking unsatisfactory right now, or your year-end projections are unsatisfactory. What should you do? Firstly, check the data to find out why things are off plan. If there is a good clinical reason, for instance to do with volume of admissions, you will need to discuss this promptly with the chief executive and/or director of finance to agree a way for handling the problem. Simply stopping elective admissions towards year-end is a primitive and unsatisfactory response and only saves significant quantities of money if beds are closed and staff levels reduced. If the problem is not admissions, the causes of an overspend are sometimes due to clinical behaviour, quirky changes in bed occupancy or drug use for instance. More often, the problem is agency staff or locum use, or overtime. The difficulty with all overspends on staff (who are likely to account for 70% of your budget) is the lag time in getting control of expenditure, either by reducing or increasing numbers, or by doing away with the need for agencies and locum staff. This is caused by the cost and clumsiness of personnel processes. You need, therefore, to keep ahead of the game and to make sure that the agreed and funded establishment is realistic and sufficient to cover leave, etc.

Changing team behaviour at short notice is difficult, often impossible, and so, boring and nannyish as it may seem to clinicians, regular briefings about the state of the budget and exhortations to prudence are as important as any specific measures.

If things are uncorrectably overspent, there may be grounds for the use of contingency funds. How best this should be arranged is debatable. Personally we favour a situation whereby the director of finance holds the contingency reserves and doles them out meanly, grudgingly, and only after the most persuasive arguments are put to him.

Capital management

Quite small directorates will have capital projects, even if they are only for the replacement of equipment. The processes by which trusts obtain capital is complex and outside the scope of this chapter, nevertheless it is important to realise that a finite amount of capital is available to a trust. This will comprise "minor block capital" for the routine replacement of equipment, etc, and may also contain funding for larger capital items. Within a trust, bids for capital will always exceed the amount available and all medical managers need to understand the local process and timetable for bidding for capital. However that process is to be undertaken, a proven business case may need to be made for anything large or new, and that business case may need to include an option appraisal—one of the options always being that no capital is made available. Details of the business planning process are included in the next section.

One of the proposed benefits of the new "Foundation" status which some well-behaved trusts may achieve is the easier access to capital and the option to borrow money for capital projects in the open market.

Conclusion

There is nothing scary about holding a budget if the process is managed competently by all parties and if you have a good working relationship with your department of finance. What is scary is an inappropriately set budget which leaves you with an impossible target, or incorrect or incomplete data which leaves you uncertain as to what is actually happening.

3.6 Business planning

I keep six honest serving men,
they taught me all I knew;
Their names are What and Why and When
And How and Where and Who.

(Rudyard Kipling, *The Elephant's Child*)

No book on management is complete without a section on business planning and no business is complete without planning, yet "business planning" as an activity is the *bête noire* of managers and for many clinicians it is the managerial straitjacket formalised into print. By contrast, clinical trainees looking towards an impending interview may see it as the one bit of the managerial mystique which they need to understand.

What does business planning mean? Simply, it implies not just thought, research, and debate about the future of the business but, crucially, the ability to distil the conclusions into a single document to which the business should work in the succeeding year or longer.

For medical managers we can usefully divide business planning into three groups of activities:

- the corporate plan
- the directorate plan
- the business plan for a specific project.

The corporate plan

The corporate plan is the all-embracing plan that trusts are required to produce each year. It must incorporate the plans of all the individual directorates, reflect purchasers' intentions, respond to general changes in the NHS, and include a response to major budget changes. Corporate plans are not produced in one sweep but evolve slowly over a year or more. The outlines that will eventually form the final business plan are the agendas for negotiations with primary care trusts and health authorities. As well as setting corporate priorities they are the starting point for directorate business plans. During the evolution of the corporate business plan there may be as many as a dozen timetabled review points when, for example, purchasers' intentions are circulated, prices decided, formal reviews of directorate plans undertaken and, finally, the point when the business plan is signed off. Details of such a process are outside the scope of this book, they are all very time consuming and not for the fainthearted. The average medical manager needs to know about the simpler but similarly structured construction of a directorate plan and to help achieve this the manager's trust should circulate explicit guidelines.

The directorate plan

The making of a directorate's business plan is not an esoteric activity. It is a simple exercise in common sense. The more down to earth it is the more credible it will be. The pulling together of the written business plan requires first that you do your planning properly; you are not simply reacting to a checklist sent down from the chief executive's office—or you shouldn't be. You should nevertheless have the list of corporate objectives in your hand when you start your own planning process. This is the "top down" planning document. What you need to add is your "bottom up" planning insights. Top down and bottom up should meet harmoniously in your final document.

The planning process at its simplest requires you to answer some questions.

For what length of time are we planning?

The time is usually one year, but with a two- to three-year horizon against which to make longer-term plans. Ten-year plans are not really worth making because they are usually overtaken by unpredictable events.

What do we want to do?

This is the bottom-up part. This can only be derived from a proper knowledge of the directorate's work. Is there some new skill the team wishes to deploy? Do they want to start an innovative type of clinic? Do you want to swap from inpatient to day care? Do you wish to appoint an extra consultant and so on.

What do others want us to do?

This is the top-down bit that requires that you know the corporate strategy. This may be a major change of service, for example, transferring radiotherapy to another trust or a response to a national initiative, such as setting a firm target for outpatient waiting times, which you will be expected to meet regardless of where it might come in your own hierarchy of targets. Additionally you will need to review messages from purchasers about what they want, from GPs, from patients (if you know), and from other directorates. These last are not really top down plans, more "sideways across" plans, but that is not proper management speak!

What is the probable budget?

It would be nice if that did not appear so soon in the list, and in traditional business planning texts it does not, but within the NHS it will invariably be a major issue so it should not be left out of the reckoning for too long. I have seen too many NHS trust corporate business planning documents full of fine words about the extra things that need to be done, followed with barely a blink by detailed sums of expected reductions in budget, sometimes frankly put, sometimes dressed up as "cash releasing efficiency savings" to make you feel better about it. Either way it may clip the wings of your grand plans early.

How do we integrate these demands?

How do we integrate the demands of others with our own and turn them into an *achievable* and *affordable* set of objectives? To answer this takes time and consultation, brainstorming sessions, discussion papers, and meetings. The solutions that you come up with need to be accepted by the bulk of the team within your directorate and their *ownership* of the final plan is crucial.

What resources will we need?

You will, in part, have answered this when refining your options, but now is the time to be more explicit about:

- finance and the sources of it
- staff—do we need more or less? Will they have different roles? Be of different grades? And if we are in need of new staff what are the recruitment plans?
- beds
- theatres
- services from other directorates, etc.

What will be the effect on other directorates?

Will closing, expanding or moving of a service completely undermine the functions of another directorate? Will we need more *x* ray or pathology tests. Have we costed them? Can the relevant directorate provide them and at the cost we expect? In dealing with this last issue you need to understand the stepwise progression that characterises the enlargement of many NHS facilities. You can understand this most easily perhaps in relation to ordering tests. It may be that the pathology department's machines, and the staff who look after them, are not currently working to capacity. Extra tests may therefore be done at a small incremental cost. However, your extra demands may require them to purchase a new machine and possibly even employ more staff. This can dramatically alter the cost of your proposals.

Most business plans undertaken by directorates have a habit of neglecting a large number of extra costs incurred by other directorates—simple things like extra meals and transport costs for patients.

Now you are just about in a position to write your business plan. Firstly though, get out last year's plan!

Writing the business plan

This is one person's job. Not necessarily the most senior in the directorate but someone who from the outset of the process has kept in their hands all the threads that must be drawn together to make the plan. This will mean getting hold of data, retaining the papers etc, keeping a record of internal decisions. The business plan itself has for some reason developed a standard format, but I do not see why you need to stick to that. For a start it traditionally begins with a "mission statement". I have a serious allergy to these and I am not alone in that, the phrase was seventh in the list of words that *BMJ* readers wanted banned. Mission statements tend to state the obvious, which in itself does no harm and can act as a gate through which all business proposals must pass, but to readers of any intelligence they are an irritation and may well discourage them from taking the remainder of the document seriously. For example, the following was proposed as an example of a medical directorate's mission statement.[13]

The Medical Directorate aims to provide high quality medical care in a cost efficient manner. It seeks to provide equal access to its services, will ensure the privacy and dignity of its patients, and will promote the wellbeing of its workforce. It will support research and education and seeks to gain a reputation for outstanding clinical practice.

This, the authors imply, will be memorable and positive and act as a "focus and inspiration for the Directorate". I submit that the average professional doctor and nurse or other in the directorate reading that mission statement might reply "What the hell do you think we are already doing? Are you suggesting that we currently don't do these things?" The answer of course may be "Yes, we are suggesting you are not doing them", but there are subtler ways of doing it. I have heard angry responses to mission statements so many times and constructive responses so rarely that one wonders why managers insist on continuing with this amateurish spin doctoring. The most effective criticism is a practical one. The problem with fine words and heroic sentiments (fuzz and bullshit) is that they rarely point to any obvious action plan, so let us hope you have, instead of a mission statement, a down to earth ten-line introduction to your business plan saying what you wish to achieve. This is the same sort of statement that you would put at the beginning of a paper that you submit to a journal. The rest of the plan is not particularly contentious and a typical business plan might go as follows.

- *Summary introduction.*
- *Current position in relation to*—long-term strategy. Redefine it. Is it still appropriate? How do directorate and corporate plans link in and then add some guesswork about future changes that will affect the directorate, new technology, and so on.
- *Last year's business plan*—how did we do? (be honest). What went well, what went badly, what are the messages for this year?
- *A brief SWOT analysis in relation to the options which might be in your new plan* (SWOT = Strengths, Weaknesses, Opportunities, Threats analysis)—for example: strength, we have a large number of diabetic patients; weakness, we do not have a good ophthalmic service dealing with diabetic retinopathy; opportunity, we are about to appoint a new ophthalmologist. This could be one of their special interests; threats, we will need extra laser equipment for which we do not have provision in the budget. Additionally, the trust down the road has just bought this equipment.
- *The proposed tactical plan*—this identifies how you are going to get on with your core business more efficiently and with better quality, and it also looks at your tactics for any new developments which you might wish to establish, for example your diabetic retinopathy service. When writing that plan you need to identify *who* carries responsibility for achieving each tactical move, *what resources* will be needed, and *what the timetable is*. Remember to include plans for communicating intentions and for training in relation to any change. Lastly, it is prudent to spell out contingency arrangements if slippage occurs in the implementation of the plan.
- *Proposals for assessment*—what are the endpoints you hope to achieve? How and when are you going to measure them? Who will be responsible for that? In what format will those measurements be delivered?
- *Data underpinning all of the above*—this is financial and activity data, etc, with contextual papers such as purchasers' intentions, corporate budget, NHS targets, and so on. Enough data should be in your plan for an

independent assessor to make a judgment about the plan. This is no different from writing a scientific paper, where you must present the data to justify your conclusions. The data in this instance may most easily be presented as an appendix.

- *Presentation of the plan*—most of the value in the business planning process is in having to undergo the discipline of arriving at the point when you can write the plan clarifying your direction. But you will of course also need to communicate the decisions, so you need a full-length business plan replete with data and appendices for people who will know what they are looking at. Even so, advice is that such a document should not exceed 20 pages. You will need a shorter, more easily readable version for communicating your plans outside the directorate and crucially to each member of the team inside the directorate.

I have used as a model the annual business plan for a directorate, but for many clinical directors their most considered planning will be directed to a specific service improvement or training issue. This may seem much more important to them than the annual business plan. The planning processes should, however, be much the same but it needs to lead to a crisper document. Clinicians who come to you with bright, innovative ideas (in truth or in their imaginations) often resent being asked to turn it into a business plan and present it to you formally. They may need to be offered expert managerial help in preparation of the document but a plan is needed.

Curiously, some NHS projects do not seem to be subject to the rigours of a proper business case analysis before being sent down the line for implementation. Where so-called "cost neutral" but obviously costly projects are wished on to you it is important to make your own realistic business case assessment early on in the process. A classic case of the inadequately funded initiative to emerge was the "Calman Plan", the revised training scheme for specialist registrars. I have seen two excellent, crisp business planning assessments of the implications of implementing the Calman proposals. The preamble listed the nitty-gritty of what the proposals required of the trust, defined the strategy for dealing with those proposals, then put them in the context of other initiatives underway, analysed the resources needed and the changed practice that could be expected, and, lastly, identified the costs in detail. These came out at between £600 000 and £1 million per trust. When undertaking this kind of "defensive" business planning, the process needs to be just as rigorous as when you are the initiator.

The other view

The other view of business planning is that it has become a sterile, cultural ritual in the world of management and that it not only wastes time and stultifies fluidity, but it rarely encourages real change. The changes which can evolve within a properly managed unit may do so without formal planning processes and indeed may happen more efficiently and more quickly. They may do this because a business plan tends to be budget-driven and by its sheer ponderousness can crush many initiatives at birth.

The cynical and more practical criticism of business plans is that no one reads them and that that does not matter because what they outline rarely happens. (The possible causal relationship between these two events often eludes the complainant.)

Despite this, we really cannot claim to be managing an NHS if we do not sign up to an intellectually credible planning process. Without it the business of management runs a risk of being static or merely reactive and has no route by which to escape the bondage of short-term constraints. However, do not forget that any business plan, to be acceptable amongst sceptical clinicians, must be:

- relevant
- explicit
- achievable
- affordable
- measurable
- and, most crucially, owned.

In fact a good NHS business plan is the mechanism by which clinicians can be drawn into involvement in the planning process.

3.7 Managing for quality

Quality in business is the way to success and fortune.

The only business goal of substance is the pursuit of quality.[14]

In the NHS quality is an unregarded poor relation. If you ask NHS staff what they are doing to improve the quality of the service you are likely to be met by incomprehension, for it is too often assumed that everybody is doing their best and that any failures of quality are failures of funding or of the way the organisation works.

What is quality?

Properly, quality of medical care should be about clinical outcomes; in essence "was the patient's presenting problem made better or improved, with the minimum of harm along the way?" But outcomes are very difficult to assess accurately and it is more normal, as we shall see later, to look at the *process* of care rather than the clinical *results* of the care. High-quality *processes* may indeed be a surrogate for quality of outcome, but the danger is that these are simply changes which improve the smoothness of the process. They appeal more to the politics of gesture and are more immediately comprehensible to patients, so they may attract more attention than those which genuinely influence the outcome. It will always be exceptionally difficult to assess the *quality* of a health service as a global attribute because quality is a product of so many things, often evanescent and only distantly related to the end product, health. How long you are in the waiting room before your first consultation about your diabetes is only remotely associated with how well you can see ten years later because of diabetic retinopathy. A classic example of focusing on the wrong part of the quality chain is the "two-week wait" initiative. Of course, in quality terms, a two-week wait is better than four, but the way it has been imposed has been expensive, frustrating and, ironically, counterproductive in that the *average* wait for new breast cancer patients to be seen in some areas has been lengthened because the option of local clinicians to make clinical judgments about the urgency of a particular patient has been subverted by a heavily and bureaucratically managed set of imposed standards. Nevertheless, the assumption that nothing can be done to improve quality in the NHS is clearly erroneous, but it is deep rooted and the first step must be to move it up the agenda.

It also needs to be remembered that there is more to "quality" in health care than the patients' experience of their treatment; there are also issues about access and equality which are as important as process and outcome.

The disregard of quality

In the NHS the reasons why an obsession with quality is not high on the agenda might be summarised as follows.

- Improved quality does not impinge on the success of the business even though the competition between providers envisaged by the Thatcher government reforms was intended to achieve this. As a business objective it has always taken third place to productivity and cost effectiveness in spite of government protestations to the contrary.
- No one loses their job if quality is consistently poor.
- There is little consumer pressure to increase quality and what there is is directed to headline topics, such as single-sex wards. What pressure there is is weak and often misdirected.
- The resources needed to improve quality are only rarely available and the exhortation that quality improvements do not imply the spending of money is perceived as false by those working in the service.
- In a conservative service, familiar only with incremental change, the radical changes needed to improve quality may simply demand too much time and effort from staff to get started.
- There are no reliable comparators to show where quality is poor. Current attempts at categorising quality through hospital "league tables", although well meaning, is crude and is not coupled with the structural changes that would allow patients to act on the information—even if it were accurate.
- Although many official *pronouncements* speak of the need to bend the service to the needs of its customers, the patients, official *actions* are likely to show that the true customers being served are the taxpayers.

Thus, moves towards improved quality are occurring against the grain of the primary activities of the organisation, and the pressures to improve quality are normally simply a matter of professional pride to the workers in the NHS, rather than the result of a concerted and managerial effort.

As if to confirm this, "quality" is often relegated to a non-mainstream department run by nurses with little or no input from clinicians and other professional groups. The role of clinical governance in raising the quality of clinical care has, nevertheless, moved the topic up the agenda and begun to involve more clinicians.

The cynic may slyly observe that a central government's demands for quality are often simply a pre-emptive defensive ploy to minimise the damage done by concurrent exercises in productivity and cost control. That aside, there is still an enormous amount that clinician managers could and should do to improve quality. However, in so doing, they need not read the copious management texts that exist on the subject; these publications first sprang from a different world when American businesses were trying to work out why Japanese products were overtaking theirs. A few concepts are transferable, but all you really need to do is to make an honest appraisal of the altogether more complicated world of health care at your door, most of whose priorities have nothing to do with the world of commerce. Patients are emphatically not customers. As a friend of mine who has spent much of the last 30 years in and out of hospital once said:

I only ask three things of the Health system. Professionalism, Compassion, and Privacy.

(J Parker, personal communication)

Traditional quality arrangements in the NHS

It has always been assumed that a quality service will be delivered by the professionals within the service as an automatic byproduct of the fact that they are professionals. This has led to individual professional groups taking responsibility for the quality of their own service. The doctors' professional performance is regulated by professionals groups, Royal Colleges, the General Medical Council (GMC) and informed by other initiatives such as the Confidential Enquiry into Perioperative

Deaths (CEPOD). The internal track record is scrutinised through clinical audit. The nurses traditionally had matron, that stickler for quality in dress standards and the details of nursing care. Physiotherapists, speech therapists, radiographers, medical physicists, etc all have their quality assurance programmes. It is fashionable to assume that this process is archaic and unable to deliver quality. In fact, these internal professional processes have quietly catalysed progressive increments in the quality of care for generations. Recently one might have noted that the CEPOD was a joint initiative by the surgeons and the anaesthetists; that the improvements in nursing education and practice and the development of the nurse practitioner grade were orchestrated by nursing organisations. The whole exercise of audit and evidence-based medicine (EBM) is not a product of the government and the NHS Executive; they merely jumped on to the bandwagon when it was already moving, coshed the driver and claimed it as theirs. What is new is the perception of central government that professional organisations and indeed professionals themselves are irremediably incapable of delivering the sort of quality that patients are perceived as demanding and that the remedy to this is to define and police a list of standards that must be achieved. Many of these standards look good in the papers but have little or no bearing on clinical outcome. The combining of these standards into "league tables" and "star ratings" is a further distraction and irritation. Clinical directors, as in so many things, will just find themselves as "pigs in the middle" again here as they try to persuade managers that targets usually have resource implications and persuade staff to put the targeted item further up the agenda than other clinically more pressing items. Managers with no experience of the private sector might usefully reflect that professionals who are dubbed the purveyors of poor quality in the NHS are capable of achieving high quality in the context of private medicine— largely because they have access to sufficient time, personnel, and resources rather than the element of personal reward.

Achieving quality improvement

Clinical quality

Since it must be health outcomes that primarily interest us as clinical managers, the first concern must be with ensuring high quality of clinical care. Although this is primarily the personal responsibility of clinicians and other professionals, it can be facilitated by management processes.

- Ensuring that professionals are properly supported within the organisation and have the facilities with which to do their jobs.
- Ensuring that appropriate people are appointed.
- Ensuring that supervision is adequate and delegation appropriate.
- Ensuring that continuing medical education occurs and that the correct amounts of study and professional leave are taken.
- Ensuring that audit is taking place regularly and effectively.
- Ensuring that agreed protocols are adhered to.
- Ensuring that the job plans are correct for the organisation's needs and that they are adhered to.

There is also the more proactive and general obligation to help the organisation work clinically in the most effective way.

One might reasonably add that one must also *reward* the achievement of quality. The award of various prizes, certificates and King's Fund recognitions are all welcome steps in this direction, but more important is giving local publicity and praise for quality improvements when they are achieved.

Risk management

In addition to normal clinical issues there are risk management issues that have a significant impact on clinical outcome, in particularly:

- the proper supervision of junior staff
- ensuring continuity of clinical care with proper reporting mechanisms between staff
- working to ensure that where necessary competent locums are appointed and proper induction procedures are in place for them.

Risk management is dealt with in greater detail in Section 6.5, "Risk and risk management".

Process improvement

Some quality improvements are dependent on changes in process that need to be both radical and extensive, that is, stretching along much of the path that the patient takes through the health system. (It is currently trendy to talk about the "patient's journey" as if this had just been invented.) This is only one of many options for quality improvement, but it depends on the contiguous implementation of changes by different teams, thus the medical manager has a central coordinating role to play in commissioning and achieving the improvement.[15] Until recently it was assumed that patients had no role to play in this, but it is welcome that even government spokespeople now admit that patients themselves have obligations and responsibilities concerning communication, attendance, and their attitude to staff.

By becoming involved in radical quality improvement measures, clinical managers are sure to brush with professional process improvement people. They need to be aware that, as in EBM and audit, there is a degree of zealatory in them that they may find irritating. If clinical managers read the papers or attend meetings they will need only to strip out what is useful without feeling the need to swallow the whole package. Process improvement has become something of an industry, taking its origins from various management fads of the 1970s, 1980s, and 1990s: total quality management (TQM); continuous quality improvement (CQI); business process re-engineering (BPR); service quality improvement programmes (SQIP), etc. You will be told that they are all very different, but in reality they are all much the same. In the NHS they differ from industry and commerce where they have notoriously been mixed in with "business re-engineering" simply as a vehicle for reducing the size of the workforce. This facet of re-engineering has led to its rebuttal as a business process, but does not mean that there are no lessons to learn from it for the NHS. In recent years the NHS has broken away somewhat from aping current business fads and packaged its own quality improvement programmes in the "clinical governance" wrapping. When *The NHS Plan* talks about "modernisation" it is, in fact, simply talking about re-engineering again but uses different jargon and some more explicit endpoints.

Regardless of what name is currently in favour for it the messages about process improvement may be summarised as follows.

- The process of health care is currently characterised by good people working in a bad system, not vice versa. More than that the system may be so inept that it requires the heroic efforts of outstanding people in order simply to function.
- A system will deliver no more than it is designed to and if a system is flawed it will go wrong regularly.
- If you put pressure on a bad system to work better you simply demoralise the people in it and may produce even more problems.
- Incremental change and "sticking plaster solutions" are not the way to improve the system; it needs redesign.
- A large improvement in quality can be achieved through radical changes in process.

At the working level the NHS exists as parallel functional units, for example facilities, medical directorates, surgical directorates, pathology services, etc and, at one stage removed, community, GP, and ambulance services. All see their own problems and try to fix them themselves. The patient's experience of the system is, however, not vertical but horizontal. Imagine "Auntie Flo" having a stroke at home and think through the units of the system that sequentially deal with her: GP—hospital switchboard—ambulance—accident and emergency department—medical directorate—stroke unit—social services—GP; and others in parallel, such as speech therapy, physiotherapy, pharmacy, radiology, and pathology. There will probably have been no formal communication between these separate units to improve the processes for the Auntie Flo's of the world; each separate unit has its own entrenched protocols, usually designed with little reference to those of others.

To rearrange the process to make it work properly needs an analysis of it that is comprehensive and made from the outside; judging the system especially from the patient's point of view. WE Deming, the father of quality improvement, talked of the need for "profound knowledge" of the system based on:

- knowledge of the system and how the parts interrelate
- knowledge of variation—understanding and measuring the causes of departure from normal so that an action can be taken

- knowledge of psychology to understand why people do what they do
- knowledge of the theory of knowledge—understanding learning processes.

This sounds rather inhibiting, as if it excluded average managers from getting started on the exercise. Average clinical managers, however, need to understand that they already carry with them an enormous supply of knowledge about clinical medicine and systems; so they are well on the road before they even start. They also need to remember that most management theory is common sense, jargonised, and that they are just as able to take the appropriate steps as highly paid professional "re-engineers". The analysis of variation merely implies a commitment to identifying the facts of variation; how often does the system not work properly and in what way? The knowledge of psychology is again a basic matter of understanding how to motivate people to embrace change. The last part, concerning the theory of knowledge, is a rather pretentious way of explaining the concept of continuous change as being a continuing learning process, in which failure is allowed to occur and the reasons both for success and for failure are analysed and built on for the next cycle of change. This is not as comfortable as falling back to the status quo when things go wrong, but is essential to the process of quality improvement. In re-engineering the danger is that you will fix on the *process* rather than the *product*, therefore when analysing the system and its failings, users (that is, staff of all grades and patients) need to be consulted. The King's Fund undertook a study of focus groups and confirmed that they do not simply ask for expensive change but tend to fix on cultural and communication issues. Setting up focus groups, however, may be difficult and it is not easy to engage ethnic minorities in them.[16]

Having re-engineered the system it is essential to revisit it regularly and to determine whether changes have had the expected results. This is the same cycle as used in audit and the same cycle as described above about learning. The diagram of the cycle is self evident, but in management books it is grandiosely entitled "The Shewhart PDCA Cycle" (Figure 3.2).

Figure 3.2 The Shewhart PDCA cycle.

The realities of process improvement

Excellence is not an act but a habit

Aristotle

Continuous process improvement is different from effective audit. In audit the actions looked at are usually small and closely defined, and acting on the results will normally only tinker with the basic process. It is the extensive, radical nature of process re-engineering which makes it difficult for the average institution. Commercial organisations can and *must* afford the huge time, cost and effort needed to re-engineer a process. Hiroshi Harade, President of the Japanese company Ricoh, quoted the cost of correcting a fault in a photocopier at the design stage as $368. To do so before shipment costs $17 000 but after the photocopier was in the hands of the customers it cost $590 000. One might think that savings in the NHS are either not there or of a totally different scale. That is true for individual trusts but may be not for the whole organisation, and the endpoint is "improved customer satisfaction" rather than a "cheaper product". Process re-engineering is time consuming and if outside consultants are brought in to help it is also very expensive. If in-house managers are used then the other work of the organisation suffers. So, contrary to the professional re-engineer's vigorous support of radical change as the means of improving quality, there is much to be said for undertaking re-engineering in bite-sized pieces—the development of one-stop clinics is a good example. You may find common factors that obstruct the development of a smooth-running service, such as archaic booking systems, difficult access to radiology, slow pathology reporting, and absent notes. A focus group of patients will identify problems that you did not know you had. These specifics need to be addressed in the first re-engineering project, but then make subsequent projects very much easier. For example, the depressing (for patients) problem of long waits and queues in outpatient departments can sometimes be tackled by the application of computerised "Decision Support Systems" which can show how best to reconfigure the booking system to avoid delays. The principles and the software are applicable in many different queuing situations.[17] The problem is that to make such an analysis, and indeed in almost all such projects, money is required at start up. The examples listed above mostly need expenditure to put them right. Enthusiasts for re-engineering say that the improvement process results in a new system which costs less to run and is more productive, although it is difficult to find examples to confirm this. The absence of start-up money has sadly led to many worthwhile projects being suffocated at birth, and is another symptom of the short-termism and compartmentalisation of NHS financing. In fairness to the ever-wary director of finance, one must add that the finances often turn out not just to be "start-up" money, and for true quality improvement a number of costs will continue. For example in my own experience on re-engineering a "one-stop clinic", it was found necessary to upgrade the salaries of the clerks to attract people of sufficient quality and to employ clinical assistants to bring down the waiting times to a manageable level. Extra equipment had to be found to enable a cytologist to work within the clinic. Most of the time and effort, however, was simply establishing written protocols and persuading colleagues in other departments to change their working practices.

The unwillingness explicitly to commit finance to projects that have quality gain rather than an identifiable health gain has tempted management to use a back-door route to quality improvement, a shabby manoeuvre all too common in the NHS. The technique is simply to demand improved quality standards as part of a purchasing process or as part of the establishment of a league table or recognition process, then to police them aggressively but not to provide any help to assist in their achievement. The purchaser–provider split and the need for service specifications has been the perfect vehicle for this kind of exercise, and as the process engineers would have predicted it often merely leads to the process corrupting itself artificially to produce the required data implying that the quality improvement has occurred when, in fact, it has not.

The manipulation of waiting lists by managers so as to achieve the demanded changes is a textbook example of this.

Quality assessment

The assessment of quality is, in essence, what audit is all about, and the definition of audit given in the "Working for Patients" White Paper of 1989 was "the systematic, critical analysis of the *quality* of medical care, including the procedures used for diagnosis and treatment, the use of resources and the resulting outcome and *quality* of life for the patient".[18] Audit will be discussed in Section 6.8, "Audit, evidence-based medicine, and managed care". What concerns us here is what quality measures medical managers can and should audit, and what are the motives for requiring them to do so. Maxwell's parameters of quality in health care mark out the areas which need to be assessed and improved: *Effectiveness, Efficiency, Appropriateness, Acceptability, Access*, and *Equity*.[19]

These are the essential contents of the clinical governance package, of which more below. Also remember that government has decided that a principle of delivering high-quality care is that these quality exercises are too important to be left to trusts and needs central support and supervision. Hence the Committee for Health Improvement (CHI), of which more later.

As *clinicians* we are concerned with the quality experienced by individual patients and are clear that quality is in two parts:

- the process should be as pleasing as possible to the patient; this is about access, communication, courtesy, privacy, environment, etc
- the outcome which should be as good as possible, that is, there should be appropriate care for maximum health gain with minimum disbenefit.

As *managers* we also wish to ensure that we are running a high-quality organisation in the business sense, optimally productive and cost effective. The assessment of business quality should not be confused with the assessment of clinical quality, and the achievement of the latter may, of course, be at the expense of the former. In commercial organisations, of course, high-quality service in the sense of process is crucial to the well being of a competitive organisation in the open market. In a normal market the pressures of consumerism are constructive. One is not supposed to mention it, but in the NHS consumerist pressures rarely focus on the real issues of health outcome, instead they may be a distraction, focusing predominantly on process and comfort issues. Thus, by using their time and energy to assess quality outcomes, medical managers need to have a clear list of priorities:

- health outcome
- process quality
- cost effectiveness.

You could argue that because poor cost effectiveness can take away money needed for achieving health gain, it should take precedence over quality of process. Either way the current problem is the obsession with measuring process quality and cost effectiveness to the exclusion of health outcome, and the problem is also to do with motive, which is as much to do with a desire for control as a desire to improve. Medical managers may also find irritating the insistence on continuous monitoring rather than on sampling, even though the continuous monitoring of data is expensive of resources and frustrating for staff. Unfortunately, the monitoring of health outcome is the most difficult.

Monitoring health outcomes

This does not mean that only endpoints need to be measured. If quality control exercises improve the accuracy of cervical cytology or mammography or reduce infection or the need for readmissions, it is reasonable to assume that there is an effect on the all-important health gain endpoint.

> Everyone wants information on clinical outcomes. These measures have an intuitive appeal: high-quality care should be reflected by good outcomes, therefore poorer outcomes should indicate deficiencies in care, including missed opportunities or wasted resources. The hope is that data on outcomes will provide a barometer for health care, indicating the effectiveness and efficiency of service delivery.[20]

However, the measurement of clinical outcome is a very inexact science. Unfortunately, some measures can be deceptively informative. Even the easiest outcome to measure, death, the number of patients having treatment who die, is only meaningful when compared to an exactly comparable population. The effects of case mix routinely frustrate interpretation, except in rare instances of sophisticated systems, such as those used for predicting the survival of ITU patients. Studies on treatments that are, or could be, multimodal show that even quite wide ranges of quality in the application of these treatments have minimal effects on measurable outcome in the short term.[21] Purchasers' measures of effectiveness and government league tables which ignore case mix and statistics are worse than useless, giving spurious honour to those whom population bias, case selection and statistical serendipity have thrust to the top of the list. For the government so often to use meaningless "league tables" in a widely publicised "naming and shaming" exercise is not simply an unfortunate reflection on their intellectual credulity but a tragedy when all it does is seed widespread anxiety into the very populations for whom they are claiming to act.

The publication of league tables does, however, change behaviour, although it may not do so in the way intended. When some states in the USA published death rates after cardiac surgery some surgeons with poor outcomes and low operating volumes stopped operating but few other changes in practice or outcome were noted. However, it became more difficult to get poor-risk patients operated upon and the database changed as more attention was paid to recording comorbidity, etc.[22] The same response is probably now underway in the UK. It is a statistical minefield fit only for trained public health clinicians, it is not what it is at present, a playground for politicians. One hopes that the interpolation of clinical "czars" to plan and monitor quality improvements may add the necessary insulation between politicians' aspirations and clinical reality. Public health doctors are well aware of the difficulties in the process of establishing clinical effectiveness indicators. The first stab at this activity produced an odd-looking list of 14 indicators, which included the obvious candidates, such as MMR in immunisation rates and breast and cervical screening coverage. The list also included quirky things like prescribing statins in general practice, for which there was no agreed standard, cochlear implant rates where the numbers are so small as to be statistically meaningless, and hip and knee replacements where previous good performance produces spuriously "poor" performance. But never mind, as long as we all keep a sense of clinical and statistical reality about us the process will be valuable quite apart from providing a lifetime of gainful employment for public health physicians.

For the moment it is a fact of life that the measurement of process is usually our best mechanism for predicting rather than measuring outcome and thus quality of care, but it does require that we measure quality by degree of adherence to very clearly defined and agreed standards. Unfortunately, these are only available in a limited number of clinical instances. For example, the percentage of premenopausal women with node-positive breast cancer receiving chemotherapy or the percentage of patients with myocardial infarction receiving thrombolysis within a set time. Medical managers need to make clear judgments about the validity of the criteria that are going to be used as "gold standards" of quality. This in turn leads back not only to the validity of EBM as a process but also to an awareness that bureaucratisation of the process can lead to the original measure being misrepresented or inappropriate. For example, concerning the management of breast cancer, when breast conserving surgery is used, a second re-excision of the area surrounding the tumour may be needed to achieve "clear margins". Recently, quality assessment questionnaires have asked for the percentage of reoperative specimens containing residual tumour. These answers are uninterpretable without a knowledge of other variables about the patient which are not collected. Furthermore, the question itself is predicated on the assumption that clear margins are essential, a view not supported by all the data. In this example a simple bureaucratic mechanism has attempted to distil a very complex clinical process and in doing so has lost its power. A powerful and valid test is one in which many questions are proposed, answers received in a pilot study are correlated with the desired endpoint—in this case quality—and then only those questions which correlated closely are asked in future. This is a technique familiar to psychologists but an alien concept it seems to many managers. In the case of poor-quality breast surgery we know the features of those surgeons and centres who have been shown to have poor outcomes.[23,24] The two main correlates are, firstly, seeing only a few patients and, secondly, having no regular contact with medical oncologists. The enthusiasts for collecting every tiny bit of data about breast surgical services need to prove that they can do better than simply acting on those two pieces of relevant data. Collecting data is of course infinitely easier than acting on it.

There are many dangers inherent in these extensive data collection processes. The first, and rarely tested, criticism is that they are simply not a cost-effective addition to our means of improving people's health. Secondly, when data collection is inflicted on people who do not themselves need it, and do not respect the motives of those who demand it, the data are unlikely to be valid. Worse than that, new forms of defensive medicine develop. The rejection of poor-risk patients is a serious but probably overemphasised example of this. A more classic example is the "Hello Nurse" in the accident and emergency department—employed solely to greet and quickly assess the patients as they come through the door in order that all patients can be said, for the purposes of quality standards, to have been assessed within five minutes. In reality, most will then wait just as long as they ever did to be properly assessed or treated.

The tragedy of the obsession with monitoring is that it is a declaration of failure. We should be expending our efforts on picking, training, supporting, and rewarding people so that we do not have to monitor their performance all the time. This is not Utopian, it is simply a different philosophy about managing of people and processes.

It has been claimed that there is a pervading culture that "Quality is asserted not measured".[25] We do need "quality control" but it must involve:

- parameters agreed by all parties as meaningful, one should be sure to avoid "The MacNamara Fallacy", so we must seek to measure what is important not make important what we can measure
- parameters agreed by all parties as useful
- measurable parameters
- parameters assessable by sampling rather than continuous measurement
- accepting that professionals within the service will act professionally
- a guarantee that data are not used out of context.

3.8 Clinical governance

The 1997 White Paper, *The New NHS, Modern and Dependable*, identified an area for attention that it called "clinical governance", which is a term whose interpretation is of the government's own making for the words themselves tell us nothing much. *Governance* can mean either "the act of governing" or "the state of being governed",[26] but the new phrase is all about maintaining standards, improving quality of care, and in the NHS appears to mean a process driven from above whereby all the threads that contribute to quality of care are drawn together in the organisation, facilitated, monitored, and policed. Nationally, a number of special forces deployed by the NHS are there to define and police the details of the process. The most important for you as a clinical manager is the Commission for Health Improvement (CHI), subsequently transmogrified into CHAI to incorporate Audit. (The original acronym was CHIMP but this was abandoned as lacking the necessary *gravitas*.) The National Institute for Clinical Excellence (NICE) critically assesses new and established treatments and decides which the NHS ought to support, but more of that in Section 6.3, "Rationing".[27] The National Care Standards Committee (NCSC) checks that private medical facilities are up to standard and the National Clinical Assessment Authority (NCAA) and National Patient Safety Agency (NPSA) try to protect patients from errors.

All trusts need a single person at board level (normally the medical director) to take responsibility for overseeing a systematic process of clinical governance that will:

- ensure continuous improvement in the quality of professional and clinical services provided by the organisation
- encourage and guide the dissemination of good practice
- evaluate, support, and monitor clinical practice
- facilitate the rapid detection and open investigation of adverse incidents and ensure that lessons are learnt from them.

The principle is worthy; the need, I suppose, self evident, although it is yet another instance of an official belief that professionals are incapable of fulfilling these tasks themselves and must be chivvied into them. Nobody really knows whether the effort that is required is justified. In management parlance will history show any "added value" or will it be perceived as just a further extension of the existing bureaucracy?

The spectrum of activities that need to be tied together is daunting. It includes quality initiatives, risk management, audit,

EBM, educational strategies, new technology, introduction of new drugs, continuing professional development (CPD), continuous medical education (CME), compliance with the European working time Directive, accreditation, complaints, poor performance enquiries, and so on. More things are photocopied, more committees redigest regurgitated products of other digestions, more and more convoluted guidance documents are issued and, unless the process is carried out extremely sensitively, those in the front line will feel undermined and untrusted and the process will be seen simply as a political exercise and another facet of the central obsession with control in the NHS.

If the process is managed delicately it may indeed help professionals to "do the right thing" and "do it the right way", and if it is to be handled well, both medical and clinical directors need to be deeply involved.

What will medical managers need to do?

When the grim-faced person from CHAI comes to visit the Medical Director of Slapdash and Poorly Health Trust as the first phase of an inspection, he or she will probably be wanting to know something which the board of any trust should already know.

- Are you ensuring that your organisation is using best practice?
- Are you educating your staff to achieve that?
- Are you monitoring your outcomes to ensure that they are satisfactory?
- Do you have the right culture and procedures to ensure that you respond promptly to anxieties about poor performance?
- Are complaints dealt with correctly and the lessons from them spread through the organisation to encourage appropriate changes in practice?
- Do you have a formal structure in place for assessing and minimising clinical risk and is there a critical incident reporting system in place?
- Do you have a means of exploring opportunities for quality improvement in different service areas?

Keeping your organisation up to standard with its clinical governance obligations needs considerable and consistent clinical and managerial input. As much of the activity is simply monitoring what is happening you may be very tempted to give the issue very low priority, but you should not. The unhappy saga of the bad results from paediatric cardiac surgical care at Bristol which unfurled themselves across the newspapers between the autumn of 1997 and the summer of 1998 and rumbled on into the next century underlines the responsibilities that clinical managers have to act in the face of data showing poor quality. Doctors who are managers, and that included in the Bristol case the chief executive who was a doctor, were judged to be reprehensible because the data were said clearly to indicate poor performance, and yet the management side failed to act. We will never know whether the outcome would have been different if the current initiatives on clinical governance had occurred eight years ago. If the culture of an organisation is wrong it needs more than directives from the NHS Executive to put it right. If clinical managers see themselves as the agents of good quality and sound practice, rather than police guarding the trust's financial bottom line, they have nothing to fear from clinical governance.

At the end of all this one wonders if all the paperwork and the exhortations and inspection committees are not actually missing the point that the real guarantors of quality are motivated, committed, supported professionals within the service, and that much of what has happened over the last ten years has damaged rather than enhanced their motivation and commitment. But I may be wrong about that. Certainly, the new bureaucracy is here to stay and as time goes by will become more difficult to dislodge from the system, however costly and useless it proves. An account of the ludicrous burgeoning of the regulation to which any clinician may now be subjected was given by Irving Taylor, Professor of Surgery at University College London. He noted that he is subject to regulation by 24 separate bodies.[28]

Preparing for a visit from CHAI

CHAI may visit you for one of two important reasons. With luck it will simply be your turn to be inspected to ensure everything is in order; more worrying would be the other sort of visit arranged because it is clear that there are problems either with the whole organisation or a part of it, for example a pathology or radiology service, and you will all have seen the hysterical reports in the media that follow the latter type of visit. However, let us assume you are told that you are about to be the happy recipient of a visit of the first sort. Do not be lulled into thinking that because your trust is not obviously the site of a problem the visit will be more benign or less thorough. This is not like the village bobby coming around to ask some questions, taking out his/her notepad, licking his/her pencil, jotting down a few facts, and then leaving politely. No, this will be a carefully planned, extensive, thorough, and potentially revealing enquiry. It is the Detective Chief Inspector and his team who will be visiting and they will be looking under the beds and in the cupboards, taking statements from your neighbours and acquaintances, rummaging through your dustbins and carefully collating all this data on their computer to ensure no crime has been committed. They have done it before, they know all the forms of evasiveness that might be encountered, and they will probably sniff out a problem if there is one. The difference with CHAI is that it exists to help you change your ways, not to present you to some court for punishment if you have strayed.

So what to do? Firstly, chaos ensues and at this stage it is important not to let all management effort be directed to dealing with the preparations for the visit. However, these visits are complex and protracted so you will need to set up a team to collect data, liaise with CHAI, and let everyone else get on with their work. You can find out about the *modus operandi* of CHAI by consulting its website and also by looking at its reports on other hospitals. In essence what will happen is the following.

- You will need to collect for them huge amounts of raw data about your business, in both paper and electronic formats.
- You will need to let them know the names of those you do business with or might have a view. These "stakeholders" include not just obvious ones such as the local primary care trusts and universities but also groups such as patient support groups and the local ambulance services. They will all be quizzed about you.

- You will need to identify key groups of employees who may be sent questionnaires and interviewed if necessary.
- You will need to make arrangements to have parts of the organisation inspected or just observed. These visits, by the way, are not meant to be secret—they should be announced in advance.

As soon as data start to accrue it is analysed by CHAI to find the fault lines and weak spots in the organisation. Not those at which a solitary grumpy patient has pointed the finger, but things that are identified by several different types of indicator all pointing the same way. It is important to add at this point that CHAI is looking for examples of good practice as well as bad, and offers praise as well as criticism. You will have a chance to comment on its report before it is issued, but once it is on the CHAI website it is there for everyone to read.

3.9 Communicating

One of the maxims of management that is almost true is that you cannot communicate too much or too often. The single most important function of clinicians in management is as communicators. They are the two-way channel between management and clinical staff, and their grounding in patient care should also help to optimise communications the organisation has with patients. The realities of NHS medicine also involve them in communicating with the media.

Communications with colleagues

Your achievements as a practical manager and leader, and your ability to get things done, will depend on your communication skills; firstly, as a listener, and secondly, as a transmitter. You may think that the simplest way to do all this is to retreat to your office, wait for the letters and telephone calls as your input, and spend your time dictating letters, tapping out emails, and concocting position papers as your output. There is a beguiling roundness about completed papers or letters, a reassuring finality about sending emails, but there is a truly Faustian risk that the process may become an end in itself, enabling you to avoid the hard grind of personal contact. Also, it fits too easily the traditional pattern of NHS management, where many messages are sent down the line but they pass very few coming up. Within the confines of a hospital, communication is better served by face-to-face contact: don't write—visit; don't send a circular—discuss at a team meeting; don't just look at the balance sheet and the productivity graphs—go walkabout. For managers, face-to-face contact involves difficult balancing acts between listening and influencing, and between promising and refusing. Psychologists like to refer to these contacts as "transactions" and where they are in relation to conflict, they are discussed in Section 4.3, "Managing conflict", and Section 4.7, "Problems with colleagues". In more normal day-to-day transactions it is important to remember the psychologists' claim that 38% of non-technical, face-to-face messages are carried by the voice or tone inflection and 55% by outward behaviour, such as body language, dress code, and physical size. This leaves only a paltry 7% of the message to be carried by the words used. An intriguing extension of this is the finding that the likelihood of a surgeon having been sued for malpractice correlates with the tone of voice he uses when talking to patients.[29] Perhaps your communication skills would be improved by an assertiveness or communication course? However, I doubt it—communication skills seem to be inherent rather than learnt.

"Walkabout" visits to a specific area, announced or unannounced, pose an interesting range of problems. They are time consuming and they commit you to a barrage of unvalidated facts and opinions. You will probably have noticed how books for armchair travellers fix not on general descriptions of places but on quirky little observations and incidents that are felt to reveal the true character of the place. So, too, with walkabouts where the truth may sometimes be encapsulated in a chance remark from a cleaner—but beware of your own susceptibility to such persuasive vignettes and check them later against hard facts.

Team meetings with consultants have a tendency to be disappointing. Consultants are, by nature, not malleable team players, and even if they come to meetings, they have difficulty in responding as equals when nurses and junior managers are present, though one hopes that this is becoming a thing of the past.

Communication throughout the organisation

This is more difficult. Indeed, the size and mix of the audience makes it impossible to communicate equally effectively with everybody. Some managers, on the assumption that the more communicating you do the better, flood the place with paperwork, none personalised, and much of it too general to be of interest to the average reader. Doctors in particular are inundated with unsolicited paper both at home and at work, so if communications are not to end up in the wastepaper bin they need to be targeted carefully. Observations suggest that some or all of the following formats are worth considering.

- Trust-wide regular information sheets included with the medical advisory committee minutes or in payslip packets.
- Regular concise information for all staff, in newspaper format if the organisation is large enough. Modern computerised desktop publishing software make this cheap and easy. A separate paper for doctors is worthwhile; it might include impending appointments, details of new appointees, timetables of educational events, changes in service availability (for example, closure of laboratories over holidays), and "plain-speak" summaries of topics of current interest.
- Wall posters for urgent and very important issues. These can summarise the message in a couple of hundred words of large type on a sheet of A3 paper in such a way that almost everyone in the organisation can be aware of the message within the day. The wording is, of course, critical as there is no supporting literature. The message must be explicit.
- Team briefing papers. I know of one hospital which has generic summaries produced by the executive at its meetings. These are printed down one side of the page. Each directorate then adds its own comments about relevance or action plans in the broad margin before circulating photocopies to the team.
- A central reference point for the bulky and boring piles of reports and directives that reach the hospital each month from the NHS Executive, regions, Royal Colleges, and educational bodies, etc. It helps if these are properly documented and cross-referenced and summaries made available.

- In the future much more use of hospital computer systems will be made, linked to the NHS network, so as to mimic the internet. This allows access from ward terminals to national and international medical databases, to hospital protocols, clinical advice, telephone numbers, news updates, and even the house officers' handbook. This is in addition to email and access to the normal information about beds, laboratory results, etc. Soon all staff will soon be able to "surf" the hospital net to obtain all the information they need. Unfortunately, that means that they will need to know what it is they need to know!

To avoid security problems, hospital computers were not at first connected to the internet, but the NHS net now provides adequate "firewalls" to allow this, thus opening up to staff not only the oceans of information to which patients have access but also allowing them their own websites.

It is difficult to know whether to recommend the copious productions of the NHS and its agencies as models of communication. Certainly, they are professionally planned and indeed their websites, advisory documents on audit, evidence-based medicine, clinical governance, etc, are models of clear language, explicit advice, and elegant presentation. These are a marked contrast to the densely typed productions on non-glossy paper which outline new legislation. The "orange book" defining the Calman training proposals was one such example,[30] the very user unfriendliness of which must have set back the process substantially. Executive Letters, now called NHS Circulars, that direct our lives, although brief, have all the presentational charm of an EU Directive. The last lesson to learn from centrally produced documents may be seen in newsletters. There is a universal indifference about their exhortatory style, presenting only accounts of success or imagined success larded with head and shoulders photographs of smiley people we have never met, and produced on expensive, glossy paper that our unfunded, hand-illustrated, photocopied handouts to patients can never hope to match. Skim and bin them!

The volume of paperwork

In 1995, the Department of Health is estimated to have sent out:

- more than one million pages to trusts and health authorities
- more than 300 management letters
- approximately 400 other publications to health authorities
- around 200 other publications to trusts.[31]

In 1995, Stephen Dorrell, then Secretary of State, set up an investigation into the means by which this volume might be reduced. The report of that investigation[32] concluded that the problem was more widespread than the above figures suggest. The British Association of Medical Managers (BAMM) ran a parallel survey[33] and concluded that the main culprits were:

- in trusts—the business planning process
- commissioning—too many and duplicated requests for data
- centrally (the NHS Executive was the major culprit in all this)—too many directives, consultation documents, and requests for data without prioritisation or targeting
- the fact that the whole system is paper based.

The solutions proposed were clearly vehicles for clinical managers to express many of their frustrations with NHS bureaucracy. Among other things they proposed:

- improved electronic communications
- targeted mailing
- authors made to draft all communications in longhand
- nothing to be longer than one page of A4 paper
- doing away with inappropriate, repetitive, and spurious monitoring and data collection exercises
- charges for the provision of data
- halving the number of people employed by purchasers
- reducing the amount of legislation applied to the NHS
- reducing central control and increasing the autonomy of trusts.

The summary makes very cheery reading, confirming a communality of complaint among clinical directors that does not normally find a platform. The Department of Health did respond to the *Seeing the Wood, Sparing the Trees* initiative, and in 1998, changed from the habit of multiple types of management letter to a single series called "Health Service

Circulars". These are available electronically (http://www. doh.gov.uk/publications). As yet, there is not much evidence of a reduction in the quantity of paperwork issued nor can one realistically expect this for as long as the NHS remains centrally managed by design, anxious by inclination and prescriptive by habit. *Seeing the Wood, Sparing the Trees* commented that "developing a more mature relationship, based on openness and trust would be the single most important move towards minimizing bureaucracy". Sadly, the obsessively prescriptive NHS of the twenty-first century seems to be heading in the opposite direction and only the limitless publishing opportunities of the internet will save the world's forests from its profligacy.

Communicating with the public

The NHS communicates ineptly with the public. Take, for example, the public meeting. NHS trusts are required to have public meetings to present themselves and their results and these meetings can be the ultimate example of a hollow communication exercise. It has been calculated that about one in 10 000 to one in 100 000 users of services attend them, usually embittered opponents of change, local politicians, and ideological zealots. The fare is often a carefully crafted best view of the organisation's achievements and the whole event may quickly descend into farce once the questions begin. It is symbolic of the impotence of the public to challenge accountability within the NHS. Public meetings to debate changes proposed in NHS facilities are organised by the local health authority, and the difficulty here is that there are rarely two or more options, the choice between which will genuinely depend on public preference. The views of those attending the meetings and those presenting at them are equally well known and the value of the exercise very limited other than to remind participants how uncomfortable change can be. The opening of trust board meetings to the public is hardly likely *ipso facto* to change the relationships into something more constructive. Managers who manage to set up a calm, apolitical, constructive two-way communication channel with their patients will have done a great service.

Communicating through the media

There are great dangers in trying to use the media as a vehicle for manipulating rather than communicating, because it is so unpredictable and unreliable. It is, however, an unfortunate reality that the upward channels to the NHS Executive and government are so tenuous that often only pressure from the media has any effect. Health stories are part of their stock-in-trade, readily carried without much attempt at checking the facts or putting them in context, partly one suspects because of the corrupting effect of deadlines and the desire for a scoop. Bricks can indeed be made without straw if they need only last a day or two. Transparently inaccurate or overstated items display an eerie lack of basic knowledge about medicine, for example one day both the *Independent* and the *Daily Mail* announced that "Australian scientists have developed the first nano-machine which will enable doctors to provide an instant diagnosis of virtually all known diseases", and on another occasion BBC Radio 4 excitedly announced that pelvic pain was to a thing of the past as doctors had discovered how to cut the nerve that joins the womb to the brain. More subtle and more damaging is the cavalier attitude to statistics, so that for instance in 1997 the public was told that the risk of breast cancer for those on hormone replacement therapy was "2·3 times higher or more than double that of non-users". In fact, the *Lancet* article, on which that headline was based, identified the relative risk as a paltry 1·023.[34,35] If efforts are not made to counterbalance the inherent naivety and imbalance of media stories, real damage may be done to patients. For example, data from the Office of National Statistics showed an unexpected rise, of 14 000 legal abortions in 1996 in England and Wales, which was attributed to women precipitately stopping oral contraception after scare stories about the safety of oral contraceptives in 1995. However, this was an improvement on the 50 000 extra unplanned pregnancies that occurred after a similar scare story in 1969. These problems are not just the fault of the media. CP Snow's *Two Cultures and the Scientific Revolution* was published in 1959 and the gulf that it identified between science (including medical science) and the rest of the world has widened since then. Susan Okie, a medical journalist on the *Washington Post*, has written about the declining scientific literacy of journalists and the deteriorating general literacy of doctors and scientists and how this widens the communication gulf.[36] Doctors have to spend much more time learning how to explain to the media as well as to patients what they are doing. For all that, medical managers need to be practised or cautious in their dealings with the media. This is particularly so when they become embroiled with the press over an unexpected crisis. A major accident in your catchment area is simply time consuming, but an apparently straightforward clinical decision may turn into a public relations nightmare—as the infamous "Child B" case exemplified. Child B was a child under the care of the Cambridgeshire and Huntingdon Health Authority; relapsing yet again from her leukaemia she was judged not to be an appropriate candidate for a second marrow transplant. The Extra Contractual Referral was refused but the father used the willing press as the vehicle for his protest at this. The health authority and the clinicians involved were thus immediately cast as the villains, a situation difficult to retrieve even with the most practised public relations; something which most trusts simply do not have. The fact that the child did not survive the extra treatment which was eventually supplied went almost unnoticed. One option is for such trusts to use external public relations agencies giving 24-hour cover. NHS trusts have been criticised for employing public relations people, and where they function simply as salespeople for trusts in a commercial market context, one can understand that criticism. They do, however, spend more time explaining trusts' activities to local people and the press, and softening the hard edge that exists between hospitals and the world outside must surely be worthwhile.

When dealing with the media remember that analysis shows their preference for bad news stories. Negative stories about doctors currently outweigh positive ones by two to one.[37] Even when reporting research, bad news is chosen in preference to good.[38] When assessing the apparent breakdown of faith between the public and the NHS, and other institutions in our society, Onora O'Neill, in her Reith Lectures, was both explicit and articulate in identifying the role played by the media in that breakdown, pointing out that ironically the media has escaped the revolution in accountability that the rest of us have suffered whilst remaining "deeply preoccupied with others' untrustworthiness".[39]

The message for medical managers from all this is to remain watchful and wary—remember that politics as well as health are part of the witches' brew when the media spoons out a sample to taste.[40]

A useful list of "fright factors" and "media triggers" appears in Table 3.1.

Communicating information to patients

We are not good at communicating information to patients. The brevity of consultations and the persisting habits of paternalistic medicine combine with a norm that non-medical staff do not give out medical facts and leave most patients in an information desert. Under pressure from patients, things are improving and alternative sources of information on the internet are burgeoning; leaflets, books, and magazines challenge us to orchestrate the production of relevant, comprehensible, and accurate material for patients. Much of what is currently given out is of very poor quality and could be improved by adherence to checklists that may be used to enhance their quality.[41] It would be a useful but probably depressing exercise for new clinical directors to collect together examples of all the information leaflets available for patients treated in their directorates and to score them for presentation, legibility, and appropriateness. Then count up the number of clinical contact points where written information would probably be welcomed by patients but is currently not available.

In relation to the internet there is a particular urgency, as even the briefest acquaintance with the thousands of health-related websites will show much information to be inaccurate, commercial, personalised, irrelevant, out of date, or just plain weird. Entertaining, but not what is needed. One of the earliest studies of the accuracy of the internet looked at advice on managing fever in children at home. Forty-one web pages were found, but only four adhered to published guidelines.[42] We know that 60–80% of users use the internet to access health information and two-thirds of these say it had some influence on their healthcare decisions. Yet studies abound showing how inaccurate the data on the internet may be and how little patients remember about the source of the data they use.[43] Fortunately, trustworthy, good-quality websites are increasingly available and internet users are becoming less naive.

Table 3.1 "Fright factors" and "media triggers": things that are particularly likely to lead to media coverage of a medical story

Fright factors	Media triggers
Risks are generally more worrying (and less acceptable) if perceived:	A possible risk to public health is more likely to become a major story if the following are prominent or can readily be made to become so:
• To be involuntary (such as exposure to a pollutant) rather than voluntary (eg dangerous sports or smoking) • As inequitably distributed (some benefit while others suffer the consequences) • As inescapable by taking personal precautions • To arise from an unfamiliar or novel source • To result from man-made, rather than natural sources • To cause hidden and irreversible damage (eg through onset of illness many years after exposure) • To pose some particular danger to small children or pregnant women or more generally to future generations • To threaten a form of death (or illness/injury) arousing particular dread • To damage identifiable rather than anonymous victims • To be poorly understood by science • As subject to contradictory statements from responsible sources (or, even worse, from the same source)	• Questions of blame • Alleged secrets and attempted "cover-ups" • "Human interest" through identifiable heroes, villains, dupes, etc (as well as victims) • Links with existing high-profile issues (or personalities) • Conflict (including conflict between experts, and between experts and public) • Signal value: the story as a portent of further or more general ills, for example: the inadequacy of regulatory controls ("What next?") • Many people exposed to the risk even if at low levels ("if could be you!") • Strong visual impact • Sex and/or crime • Reference back to other reports the fact that something is a "story" is often itself a story, creating a snowball effect as media compete for coverage

(Reproduced from: Rodwell L. A matter of perspective. *NHS Magazine* 1998;**12**:11)

Happily, an increasing number of internet sites are now available to help website constructors, doctors, and patients through the jungle (http://www.hiquality.org.uk, http://www.resourcefulpatient.org) and there are sites recording dubious claims (http://www.quackwatch.org) and one devoted to collecting evidence of harm arising from use of advice given out through websites (http://www.medcertain.org/daeri/). The budgets needed for communications with patients have often been missing in the past, but in the future medical managers will need to make sure that not only is information made available before, during, and after people's contact with hospitals, but that information is consistent with what actually happens. The arrival of crude and potentially misleading league tables has added impetus to hospitals' need to communicate the real facts to its patients. What is intriguing is that in a world besotted with EBM, there is precious little evidence that giving patients more information so as to allow them choice is reflected in better outcomes, or indeed greater happiness.

References

1 Simpson T, Scott T. *Leading Clinical Services*. British Association of Medical Managers, 1997.
2 Council of International Hospitals. *The Role of the Clinical Director*, 1997, October.
3 Association of Trust Medical Directors. *The Role and Responsibility of the Medical Director*. British Association of Medical Managers, 1996.
4 Rivett G. *From Cradle to Grave*. London: King's Fund 1998.
5 Bradshaw A. Charting some new challenges in the art and science of nursing. *Lancet* 1998;**351**:438–40.
6 Quail M. Nurse executive's pay: a survey for the Royal College of Nursing. *Health Serv J* 1997;9 January:9.
7 Caplan RP. Stress, anxiety and depression in hospital consultants, general practitioners and senior health service managers. *BMJ* 1994;**309**:1261–3.
8 Graham J, Potts HW, Ramirez AJ. Stress and burn-out in doctors. *Lancet* 2002;**360**:1975–6.
9 Institute of Work Psychology, University of Sheffield. Cited in the *Observer*, 15 March, 1998.
10 Kent G, Johnson AG. Conflicting demands in surgical practice. *Ann R Coll Surg Engl* 1995;**77**(Suppl.):235–8.
11 Cited in "Style section". *The Sunday Times* 1997;23 March:39.
12 Howard P. *Weasel Words*. London: Hamish Hamilton, 1978.
13 Hurst DK. Business planning. In: Hurst DK, Clements RV, eds. *Clinical Director's Handbook*. London: Churchill Livingstone, 1995, p. 46.
14 Caulkin S. Interview with Stainton J. *Observer* 1997;9 October.
15 Berwick DM, Enthoven A, Bunker JP. Quality management in the NHS: the doctor's role. *BMJ* 1992;**304**:304–8.
16 Long-term Medical Conditions Alliance. *Patients Influencing Purchasers*. NHS Confederation, 1997.
17 Worthington D. Queue management. In: Cropper S, Forte P, eds. *Enhancing Health Services Management*. Milton Keynes: Open University Press, 1997, pp 177–98.

18 Department of Health. *Working for Patients*. Working Paper 6, Command 555. London: HMSO, 1989.
19 Maxwell R. Quality assessment in health. *BMJ* 1984;**288**:1470–2.
20 Davies HTO, Crombie IK. Assessing the quality of care. *BMJ* 1995;**311**:766.
21 Mant J, Hicks N. Detecting differences in quality of care; the sensitivity of measures of process and outcome in treating acute myocardial infarction. *BMJ* 1995;**311**:793–7.
22 McKee M. Indicators of poor clinical performance. *BMJ* 1997;**315**:142.
23 Salisbury R *et al.* Influence of clinician workload and patterns of treatment on survival from breast cancer. *Lancet* 1995;**354**:1265–70.
24 Gillis CR, Hole DJ. Survival outcome of care by specialist surgeons in breast cancer. *BMJ* 1996;**312**:145–7.
25 Spiers J. *The Invisible Hospital and the Secret Garden*. Oxford: Radcliffe Medical Press, 1995, p. 50.
26 *Longman's Dictionary of Contemporary English*. London: Longman, 1978.
27 Department of Health. *A First Class Service: quality in the new NHS*. Health Service Circular HSC(98) 113. London: HMSO, 1998.
28 Taylor I. Doctors' unhappiness. *BMJ* 2002;**324**:1453.
29 Ambady N, Laplante D, Nguyen T *et al.* Surgeons' tone of voice: a clue to malpractice history. *Surgery* 2002;**132**:5–9.
30 NHS Executive. *A Guide to Specialist Registrar Training*. London: Department of Health, 1995.
31 NAHAT Briefing Paper. No 99, June 1996.
32 NHS Executive. *Seeing the Wood, Sparing the Trees*. London: Department of Health, 1996.
33 Simpson J. The burden of excessive paperwork in the NHS. *Clinician in Management* 1996;**5**:5–7.
34 Horton R. ICRF from mayhem to meltdown. *Lancet* 1997;**350**:1043–4.
35 Abbasi K. Headlines: more perilous than pills. *BMJ* 1998;**316**:82.
36 Okie SM. Behind the headlines. *Harvard Med Alumni Bull* 1998;**72**:22–4.
37 Nazia Y Ali, Theobe YS, Victoria L, White PD. Bad Press for Doctors. 21 year survey of three national newspapers. *BMJ* 2001;**323**:782–3.
38 Bartlett C, Sterne J, Egger M. What is newsworthy? Longitudinal study of the reporting of medical research in two British newspapers. *BMJ* 2002; **325**:81–4.
39 O'Neill O. *A Question of Trust*. Cambridge: Cambridge University Press, 2002.
40 Fitzpatrick M. *The Tyranny of Health*. London: Routledge, 2000.
41 Jadad AR, Gagliardi A. Rating health information on the Internet: navigating to knowledge or to Babel? *Lancet* 1998;**279**:611–14.
42 Impicciatore P *et al.* Reliability of health information for the public on the World Wide Web. *BMJ* 1997;**314**:1875–81.
43 Powell JA, Darvell M, Gray JAM. The doctor, the patient and the world-wide web: how the internet is changing healthcare. *J R Soc Med* 2003;**96**: 74–6.

4: Managing people

Doctors tend to think they are good at managing people because they are doctors but it does not follow. Doctors' normal interpersonal relationships are fourfold:

- with patients
- with their teams
- with colleagues
- with friends.

The first and second are highly structured hierarchical relationships in which doctors are the acknowledged dominant partners. The third and fourth are primarily peer relationships in which the skills are social and do not much involve inspiring, leading, persuading, negotiating, managing conflict, or delegating, skills central to the management role because managers have to get things done through others.

Despite the social handicaps of their professional experience, in my experience doctors are no better and no worse than managers at deploying these special skills, which are mostly innate or learnt informally. These skills are, in fact, so difficult to teach that one needs to choose clinical managers who can come to the job with the skills in place.

Specific tasks when managing people include:

- getting the best out of people
- building a team or making appointments
- managing conflict
- dealing with contracts and job descriptions
- rewarding staff
- managing difficult colleagues
- sick doctors
- arranging and monitoring personal and professional development.

We will look at these in turn.

4.1 Getting the best out of individuals

Management texts like to start by quoting MacGregor's X and Y theories about the motivation of people at work. Theory X suggests that people are lazy, would rather not work, and will only do so when coerced. Furthermore, average individuals wish to be told what to do and, if they have personal security, will be content. Theory Y suggests that people actually find work stimulating and satisfying and have an inherent capacity to work towards objectives. Most have an untapped capacity to take the initiative with problems and be responsible for achieving targets. Individuals gain the greatest satisfaction through achieving these targets.

Management texts then suggest that there lurks a Y person in every X person, waiting to be brought out by good management. This smacks somewhat of Christian notions of original sin and the possibility of redemption through love but appeals as a modus operandi. Rather more cynically one should perhaps accept that the concepts define not just two possible types of worker but caricature two stereotypes of workers imagined by managers. Most people, of course, have a bit of theory X in them and a bit of theory Y and need to be managed accordingly in the hope of being moved entirely into the Y configuration.

Although the principles of getting the best out of people are well known and consistent through management teachings, it is sad how many people in the NHS are made unhappy not by the major and intractable problems of the service but by local irritants and bad person-to-person management. Human relationships are indeed the real tragedies of life. When managing people the touchstones of success may be to:

- include them in the team
- understand their informal cultural relationships with you and with their peers (not easy if you are a doctor)
- set them clear and achievable targets, ideally as a joint exercise
- provide constructive feedback and to recognise achievement freely
- support them in times of difficulty
- reward them appropriately
- allow them opportunities to develop new skills.

If all this is done well employees will, in theory, share the team's purpose, be loyal, motivated, and at the end of the day, content. Interestingly, financial reward is not seen to be as important in all this as you would expect. If you wish to see these truths in action in your own hospital I suggest you look at the nurses.

Nurses are a very mobile labour force familiar with voting with their feet, so you can learn a lot by finding which areas in the hospital attract nurses and which areas have high turnover and vacancy problems—then gently look for the reasons. Turnover among nursing staff each year exceeds 25% in many NHS hospitals and 65% of nurses report that they worked longer hours than they are contracted to do, much of it unpaid. But if your organisation troubles to find out from those leaving the exact reasons for their doing so (by using exit interviews or questionnaires), you will find that it is often because of:

- unachievable workloads owing to failure to set or recruit to a realistic establishment
- insufficient resources to do the job properly
- unsympathetic ward sisters or managers
- no opportunities for professional development
- they believe they have been graded unfairly.

All but one of these reasons reflect on the management skills—or lack of management skills—brought to bear on them.

Supporting staff

You can judge a company by the people it keeps.

(Advertisement for Microsoft Corporation)

If you are a clinical director or medical director you are effectively an employer in the eyes of the team and you have it in your gift to be a good employer or otherwise. This has nothing to do with your training as a manager, it is the human stance that you take and, as a doctor, a hard, financially driven attitude to your staff is less likely to be forgiven than it might be in a non-clinical manager. You will not be forgiven if in collaboration with the nurse manager you try to make savings by setting unrealistically low staffing levels or insist on inappropriate skill mixes. When managing individuals the particular areas in which your response can be kindly and humane include, in particular, sickness leave and maternity leave; both are legal, but whilst some managers are grudging about it others are sympathetic. Of course sick leave is open to abuse, and if many episodes are taken either as prolonged leave or multiple short uncertificated breaks, you may need to enquire in a more detailed way to find out what is going on. Not to do so is unfair to the person in question and to the colleagues carrying the burden of their absence. However, there are some well-trodden paths to follow in such an enquiry.

For repeated short-term absences interview the employee concerned to obtain their account of the reasons for them. You may then need to refer the employee to the occupational health department if it seems that there is genuinely a chronic health problem but beware of the multiple poorly explained absences that may represent alcohol problems. What you must *not* do when exploring the reasons for absence is to start making clinical medical judgments about employees yourself, however tempting it may be. To be frank I think the convoluted business of "absence management", except perhaps where it applies to medical staff, is not an area for clinical managers to become involved. It should be done by the personnel department with the assistance of your non-clinical manager.

Long-term sickness

Although this too should not be your business you are likely to be caught up in the process. Importantly, you will need to remember your clinical habits of caring rather than your managerial reflexes that might view such absences as a drain on resources or just as a nuisance. Make sure that:

- occupational health is involved
- the employee is being contacted regularly at home
- reintegration plans are in place for the end of the illness.

If the ill health is such that premature retirement is needed, or worse than that, the employment must be terminated, you *must* contact your personnel officer to find out how to go through these processes. They are complex and need to be handled with the utmost sensitivity. In the rare and unhappy event of serious or terminal illness in one of your employees, you may need to chase up the complex bureaucracy that surrounds early retirement on the grounds of ill health to ensure that it works speedily and humanely.

Maternity leave

Maternity leave can be a headache for you. Firstly, part of the cost may be funded from your clinical budget, and there may also be problems associated with the appointment of locums or making other arrangements. Do this early. In these situations, long-term locums are not too difficult to find but ensure that they are offered short-term contracts and try to allow a handover period. The time when the expectant mother leaves the organisation should be very predictable and she is required to give you notice of the start date of her maternity leave at least 15 weeks prior to her expected date of delivery. To be entitled to paid maternity leave she need work for the organisation for only six months so it's perfectly legal for a woman to be interviewed for a job, not to disclose that she is pregnant and then take maternity leave! So-called "ordinary maternity leave" is allowed for six months and the first six weeks are paid at 90% of her average weekly earnings; for the remainder of the six months she is paid £100 per week. At the end of her ordinary maternity leave the mother may, if she wishes, take a further six months of maternity leave but this is unpaid. Employers, including the NHS, may top up these sums to match normal pay rates for under the Employment Act 2003 fathers are entitled to two weeks' paternity leave within eight weeks of the child's birth and are paid at the lesser of £100 per week or 90% of normal weekly earnings. Fathers intending to take such leave really must be encouraged to declare it early if it is not to degenerate into episodic uncovered absences.

Returning from maternity leave may be a daunting prospect for many mothers, who in prospect thought it would be straightforward, but whose new postpartum, softer psyche sees the prospect of separation from her baby as almost intolerable. In all, 44% of new mothers do not return to work after giving birth, and 10% of these are because of lack of flexible working options. Try to help by ensuring that someone keeps in touch with the mother while she is away from work and help her to ensure that, if she wishes to return, proper creche or nursery arrangements have been made. Once the mother is back at work you will need to be sympathetic to her occasional need to arrive late, leave early, or even to be absent if her baby or babyminder is sick. Returning mothers with children under the age of six are entitled to ask to work flexibly.

Employees with at least one year's service are entitled to take up to 13 weeks' unpaid "parental leave" and this can be taken for up to five years after the date of birth or adoption. For parents of disabled children the entitlement is up to 18 weeks. Employees cannot sign away their rights under employment law so do not try to persuade them to and remember that in these matters, as in so many others relating to employment law, it is easy to fall over and land up in an employment tribunal. Acting to ensure that the service works properly so that patients are not put at risk is, in this context at least, no defence so make certain that you always refer to and defer to your personnel (human resources) department.

Too much leave

A sensitive measure of a team's performance is sickness levels. Although, of course you should be sympathetic to genuine sick leave, you need to take a hard look at the reasons for multiple leave. Find out what sort of sick leave has been taken—is it one area or ward? How does it compare with other areas of the hospital? Does it have the features of inappropriate leave, for example Fridays and Mondays, during school holidays, during prebooked annual leave, when a particular manager or ward sister is on duty, or is it during major sporting events? Any of these enquiries may point to a managerial problem. These absences may not be just laziness but are often due to features such as undermanning, leading to stress, or to a confrontational style of leadership from a manager or ward sister. Try to correct that and if an individual is at fault, once again contact the personnel department, particularly if you think formal disciplinary processes are needed as these must be done "by the book". Do not forget that all employees are entitled to a reasonable amount of unpaid leave to deal with emergencies related to their dependants.

Shrinking the team

It may be that, for whatever reason, you conclude that someone in your team has to go, be fired, outplaced, relocated, made redundant, persuaded to retire, anything! In these circumstances, and as soon as that little spark comes into your head telling you that this is the solution, *do nothing, write nothing, say nothing.* Go immediately and confess to your personnel manager, because if the processes are not completed in exactly correct detail you could find yourself in a seemingly endless spiral of appeals and tribunals that will make you wish you had never embarked on the process in the first place.

It seems extraordinary that a few years ago mechanisms were established in London (and other big cities) to cope with what was expected to be a tide of redundancies of all grades following implementation of the mergers and bed reductions recommended in the Tomlinson Report.[1] Now that we see a truer picture of what resources we need, we realise that we are in fact rather short of many staff, especially doctors and nurses, so it is rare that you will be making people redundant. Nevertheless if staff are made redundant there may be "slotting in" arrangements to enable them, for better or worse, to be accommodated in vacancies elsewhere in the organisation. If for any reason you have to make consultants redundant remember that it is prohibitively expensive to make anyone between the ages of 50 and 60 redundant (often the very person you might wish to be rid of). For those aged over 60 a negotiated early retirement is often a reasonable avenue to explore, but only after careful costing of the options by the personnel and finance departments.

4.2 Building a team

Managers and clinicians are only successful if they are part of a good team. There are many teams within a hospital—the board, the executive, clinical directorates, and smaller teams assembled for specific purposes. The physiology and pathology of such teams is a large topic, outside the scope of this book, but theory abounds and hypothetically could be used to build the perfectly effective and harmonious team.[2] Unfortunately, in most circumstances in the NHS one's options about who may be recruited to a team are limited. Indeed, as a recently appointed medical manager, you will usually come to a basic preformed team; for example, a clinical services manager, a finance manager, someone from nursing, and someone from personnel. In that sort of team at least the members are already committed to its purpose; more worrying are teams that come together in the guise of committees where the tendency is for the team to be you and your managerial helper plus one consultant, one nurse, one junior doctor, and one GP—all recruited by somebody else from a skimpy supply of volunteers.

If you do have an opportunity to put together a team yourself you should try to do the following.

- *Recruit from other than volunteers*: this may require some assiduous persuading of the "right" people. If you allow yourself to be victim of a pseudo-democratic process that simply delivers representatives to your team you may not get the skills or the commitment that you need, you may even get the opposite.
- *Try to get a functional mix of personality types*: you will, of course, make straightforward human judgments about this, but knowledge of Belbin types might help you achieve the right mix.[3] A brief summary of the Belbin types is given below.

  - the *Chairperson* presides over the team and coordinates its efforts to meet external goals and targets. They are distinguished by a preoccupation with objectives, they set the agenda, and they establish priorities.
  - the *Shaper*: just as the chairperson is the social leader, so shapers are task leaders, supplying a lot of personal input to form the application of the team's efforts.
  - the *Plant*: the ideas person, they tend to be original and radically minded; usually the most intelligent and imaginative member of the team.
  - the *Monitor/Evaluator*: this is the person who analyses and criticises the ideas that the team is working with, they are good at assessing large volumes of data and analysing this objectively.

- the *Company Worker*: the practical organiser, who takes the decisions and strategies of the group and turns them into defined and manageable tasks that people can actually get on with.
- the *Resource Investigator*: the member of the team who most easily goes outside the group to bring in new ideas; a social, gregarious team member but not a generator of original ideas.
- the *Team Worker*: the member most sensitive to the psychology of the remainder of the team; a good listener and communicator who promotes unity and harmony in the team and works to avoid confrontation.
- the *Finisher*: preoccupied with order, neatness and the completion of tasks.

It is hardly surprising that each of these characters has their own psychological type, and after many years of research Belbin was able to categorise them on the basis of their intelligence, dominance, extroversion/introversion and stability/anxiety scores.

The crucial members, too often missing, tend to be one of two types. Firstly, the *Chairperson* or *coordinator*, who sets the work of the team underway and structures that work (this should be you!). Secondly, you will find too few *finishers*; these characters are often self effacing and quiet, not advertising themselves as potential members of the team.

- *Define the overall tasks of the team and of its individuals*: these should be SMART
  - structured
  - measurable
  - achievable
  - realistic
  - timed.

In groups such as a hospital executive or a clinical directorate the tasks of a team are multiple and self evident, but a formal exercise to identify them is nevertheless necessary, and by so doing it is also crucial to define the individual roles of the specific members of the team.

Having assembled a team and defined its tasks, how do we make it work well? It is sometimes assumed that the common ideological goal of caring for patients is enough on its own to bond and motivate a multidisciplinary team, so perhaps it is not surprising how rarely anyone perceives the specific need to bond a team. All teams take time to establish themselves, members need to discover each others' personalities, work out their interpersonal difficulties, and define the group dynamics. Shared time and shared responsibilities will push a team together in due course and the clinical signs will be the appearance of "in jokes", recognised alliances, and tensions. The early stages of team development need some supervision, particularly where members of the team are seen regularly to be departing from the joint goals. Such departures should be openly aired in the group if the disruptive members are not to be left regularly disturbing business. To achieve this it is crucial that the team should have a clear mandate and corporate perspective.

"Away days" are good bonding mechanisms as long as they are planned well ahead to allow clinicians to escape from their clinical work with a good conscience. "Away days" encompass the normal bonding activities of eating and drinking together, but fortunately within the NHS we have not yet embraced the more extreme versions of this bonding activity where the team goes away to climb impossibly high mountains and swim in horribly cold lochs. I believe the evidence that such "outward bound" activities do much good is slim.

Similarly, I have never discovered whether there is any evidence as to whether the inclusion of partners (husbands, wives, *et al*) at team social occasions is beneficial or disruptive. Partners must suffer many of the unpleasant side effects of the management process at a distance: late arrivals, early departures, fallen soufflés, and missed children's parties, so they may have little sympathy for it; but they also develop a sense of curiosity about the characters that people their partners' working lives. In my experience one of the difficulties of including partners is that most management teams have a good proportion of domestically dysfunctional members, so that the inclusion of partners in any team-building activities is out of the question.

Time is in short supply in the NHS, so once you have a satisfactory team delegation becomes crucial. Of course, delegatees must understand what is expected of them over what timescale; feedback to them must be predictable and, when appropriate, congratulatory. There is a tendency in the

NHS to believe that people will do a job for its own intrinsic worth and do not require the simple reward of recognition and congratulation.

Recruitment and appointment

It cannot have escaped anyone's attention that the government has at last been persuaded of the reality that good quality can only be delivered if there are enough doctors and nurses and others to deliver it, and that in the UK the numbers of frontline staff remain wholly inadequate even though the number of doctors working in the NHS has increased by 44% in the last decade. As a medical manager one of your most specific tasks will concern recruitment and appointment, and this will affect you particularly when it concerns consultants, senior nursing, and managerial posts. In many centres you will be undertaking this in a competitive market. The recruitment of what were previously called "junior staff", PRHOs, SHOs, and SpRs may not seem to affect you much except that you need to ensure continued recognition of the posts. There is, however, a section of your workforce that needs careful handling. This is the new "lost tribe" of associate specialists, staff grade doctors, trust doctors, and "clinical fellows"—brought in primarily to help meet working hours targets and whose number has increased fourfold over the last decade.[4] These "non-consultant career grade" (NCCG) posts are a shameful reflection on our failure to handle the realities of staffing the NHS and are a potential hotbed of disaffection and resentment. Before establishing any such post you ought to consider whether another consultant, a bid for an extra, properly approved SpR post, or the reorganisation of work within the team to allow non-medically qualified people to do more might not be a better response.

Recruitment

Doctors familiar with the career structure for doctors, and mindful perhaps of their own difficulties in getting the job they wanted, may assume that recruitment simply means advertising and waiting for the replies. Nowadays, recruitment in London and other cities must be an active business as the burgeoning needs of *The NHS Plan* have led to skill shortages.

But the needs of *The NHS Plan* are only one of several reasons for this, others include:

- inadequate national workforce planning
- high dropout rate among trainees
- inappropriate limitations on some consultant-grade posts
- inflexibility and delay in granting work permits for overseas doctors.[5]

Difficulties in recruiting doctors can occur even in the most prestigious of organisations. If your hospital is not blessed by a good reputation and a nice address this may be a major issue for you and successful recruitment may even require you to change the job plan, the terms and conditions of service, or both. Even with extra effort put into recruitment, including recruitment overseas, you may still be unable to recruit and you may have to look at other ways of having the work done. In nursing the problem is worse and more worrying than it is for doctors. Although you are unlikely to be involved in the day-to-day practical chores of appointing nurses, because their turnover rate is so high that it is a full-time job, you will not escape having to deal with the consequences of the difficulties of recruitment. You will need to understand why this is more than a temporary problem and why simply increasing the effort to recruit may not be the long-term solution. Some simple facts and a basic knowledge of mathematics will suffice!

- 25% of all nurses will reach retirement age within the next 10 years. Less than 20% of registered nurses are aged under 30.
- Currently 20 000 new nurses are needed per year; by 2010 this will have risen to 25 000.
- Although the number of students enrolled in nursing courses increased from 62 000 to 117 000 between 1995 and 2000, one-third of these currently fail to register to practise at the end of their courses and 10% of those who do practise outside the NHS.
- On any day there are about 20 000 vacant nursing posts in the NHS.
- Each year 10 000 more nurses leave the nursing register than join it.
- New nursing roles outside original established positions are steadily being created.

- Nursing salaries consistently fall behind those of equivalent occupations outside the NHS.
- Increasing numbers of nurses emigrate or leave nursing.
- The number of school leavers is falling.

There are, in theory, solutions and these are apparent from other data. There are 140 000 nurses currently not working and 69% of them say that inflexibility of working hours is the major reason for this. In a Royal College of Nursing Survey, 43% of all nurses claimed to have dependent children. Although this is unsurprising, it does mean that to bring these nurses back into the workforce you will need to pay considerable attention and perhaps devote some of your budget to the provision of creche facilities, to the reorganisation of the pattern of working, and to cultural attitudes to part-time work. Nurses need to be valued more than they are at present both financially and socially.[6] As a manager you will need to address these problems, simply recruiting nurses from overseas is merely a part of the solution and a fragile one at that. All developed countries are short of nurses and quite apart from the morals of poaching nurses and doctors from developing countries the reality is that the USA and Europe are now poaching these same nurses from the UK.

The issues mentioned above may also apply to the difficulties in recruiting doctors. Currently, around 50% of medical graduates are female and the "wastage" rate is high largely because traditional forms of working and of training are incompatible with family life for those who have children. Even if medical mothers wish to return to work in due course, the system is unhelpful or frankly even obstructive. Those that stay on or return tend to do so in general practice rather than in hospital practice.

For female doctors the problems do not just concern child care facilities. They also involve part-time training and part-time working. We are very bad about facilitating this, especially in hospitals. HM (69)6 made provision for flexible training schemes for doctors, but even now only 7% of SpR and 2% of SHO posts are flexible.[7] Hospitals are unenthusiastic about taking on these trainees and there are problems with funding. Such part-time training also seems to be unpopular with trainees, quite simply because most are half time and thus only half the necessary training is achieved per year so the training needs twice as long. The unpalatability of this leads to a number of trainees having incomplete training. Such doctors can only be fitted into non-consultant-grade posts. Unfortunately, the abject resistance of the BMA to the establishment of meaningful non-consultant-grade posts has penalised people looking for part-time posts and the occupants of the posts are not a happy group. More than 50% of associate specialists are required to be involved in junior on-call rotas and few find that there are opportunities or funding for further education; almost all feel exploited. Even the term "non-career" grade has become a pejorative one, as if these doctors' commitment was less than total. As a medical manager, even without the support of the BMA, there is plenty of leeway within the current regulations to make arrangements that will attract high-quality doctors who might otherwise be lost to the system, although you will almost certainly first have to do battle with the full-timers who tend to be unsympathetic.

If you have difficulty recruiting into normal full-time house officer and SpR posts you will need to review your unit's current performance against a well-recognised list of factors which discourage trainees from looking at certain jobs:[8]

- insufficient supervision and support
- inadequate time and funding for study
- poor working environment, especially bad accommodation and inadequate provision for meals out of hours
- lack of processes for monitoring and responding to junior doctors' concerns
- failure to meet New Deal hours standards.

The same sort of issues will, of course, affect the recruitment of nurses and others. As a manager you can, in theory, act to correct problems, but I have to admit that I am not alone in having had frustrating experiences of trying to persuade managers with no experience of frontline working that abolishing or failing to maintain doctors' and nurses' residences and of making puny financial savings by abolishing proper eating facilities at night is counterproductive.

Retaining staff

In addition to the factors identified above, there are particular factors which affect the decisions of older staff about when they will retire. Now I fully appreciate that you may be aching to arrange an ill-attended leaving party for certain of your crustier and argumentative older consultants. If they want to go, have no special skills, are not fulfilling their contract, and you are sure you can replace them with keen young acolytes of yours then go ahead, let them retire. Remember though that they just might know a few things you do not and have few skills that you simply will not be able to replace. Whatever your personal attitude, the fact is that consultants, in line with most other skilled workers are seeking earlier and earlier retirement and in the NHS this trend is accelerating. In 2001 I spent an intriguing but often depressing six-month sabbatical looking at why consultants are retiring early.[9] The reasons, as you could guess, are:

- pressure of work, especially "on-call"
- stress from irreconcilable pressures asking for improved results without provision of resources
- reduced support from junior clinical and other staff
- the perceived change from a vocational, professional role to that of an abused and undervalued "process worker"
- the "hassle" factor from increased bureaucratisation and regulation
- a belief that those who retire earlier live longer.

The notion that you live longer if you retire early is, in fact, untrue; life expectancy is almost the same whether you retire at 60 or at 65. The good news for you, the clinical director who has now decided that you want curmudgeonly old Dr Grump to stay on, was the counterintuitive finding that 77% of those planning early retirement say they would stay on if an appropriate contract could be arranged. The new contract that these potential "stayers on" will want is for four to six sessions a week, with no on-call work, retaining any merit awards they have, and not predjudicing their pensions. And, by the way, most do not want to have any management sessions in their contracts, though most want to teach or mentor. In essence, they just want a clinically satisfying, hassle-free life and more time off. The DoH in its "flexing retirement" policies has embraced the acceptability of such a career change but evidence shows that it is trust human resources staff and clinical directors who are

Figure 4.1 Composite diagram of factors encouraging clinicians to retire early from the NHS.

usually lukewarm about it, probably because of the difficulties in filling what is essentially half a vacant consultant post. The reasons why people retire early are multifactorial so it is not easy to develop a reliable strategy for discouraging it (Figure 4.1).

The process of appointing staff

For the purposes of this chapter let us fix on the appointment of consultants because it will be a certain role for clinicians in management and because it is the type of appointment most beset by regulations. The process has much in common with that for other senior appointments that you might be involved with. Let us take the process step by step.

A vacancy is due

In general it is clear when a vacancy becomes due as most are consequent upon retirement. For a consultant appointment you really ought to begin the replacement process a year before the date of retirement. This is made difficult by consultants taking early retirement and being hesitant about the exact date. The first and often ignored step is openly to ask two questions.

- Do we really need to refill this post?
- If so, should it be the same job?

A retirement is a heaven-sent opportunity for change, not to be wasted. However, if after reflection a replacement is judged feasible, desirable, and is funded, you will need to concoct three documents: a job description; a job plan; and a person specification.

- *Job description*: much of this will follow a standard format (*see* Table 4.1). The personnel department will usually write this with you, as most of the items concern things such as health clearance, patient confidentiality, leave, etc.
- *Job plan*: it is important that this, like the job description, is tightly drawn. "Drift" used to be a real problem with consultant appointments. You would appoint someone to a post as a consultant geriatrician only to find them conducting interventional endoscopy, or appoint a hand surgeon to discover that no hand service had been set up but breast reconstructions were on the increase! The job plan should specify the sessions in detail. These are, of course, open to subsequent change but only by negotiation and agreement. The regional college or faculty advisor needs to ensure that it is properly balanced. The advisor has three weeks in which to comment, after that approval is assumed.
- *The person specification*: you may have seen these for jobs outside medicine:

The successful applicant will typically have 10 years' experience in worldwide dynamic marketing strategies, will be fluent in at least nine languages and have a persuasive and sunny disposition with nice white teeth—package 50–90K plus car, schooling, housing, profit-sharing scheme, and stupendously generous pension.

117

Table 4.1 Outline of the job description required for a consultant

Title of post	
Employing authority	
Place of employment	
Nature of appointment and hours of work	This explains that part-time employment is allowable
Background	This should give a snapshot of the hospital or unit and the team which the appointee will join
Overall purpose of the post	This must be very explicit and say what service the post-holder is to provide. To confirm that there is an emergency on-call rota and that cover is needed for absent colleagues on sick, annual, and study leave. That the post-holder will need to undertake teaching and to participate in administration. That the post-holder will be committed to audit and to service development
Duties and responsibilities	This enumerates the number of sessions and lays out in detail where those sessions might need to be carried out
Firm structure and support services	This will enumerate the other members of the team, secretarial support, etc
Managerial	This should outline the management structure of the unit in which the appointee will work
Health and safety	Points out the need for safe working, care of personal health and safety, and includes specifics about attendance at occupational health, for instance to check hepatitis status
Confidentiality	Outlines the organisation's duty of confidentiality to patients and might usefully add a section on an individual's right to draw attention to deficiencies in the service
Timetable	This is the job plan
Terms and conditions of service	This may point out that Whitley Council provisions apply and outlines the annual leave allowance, equal opportunities regulations, superannuation, removal expenses, etc

It is not like that in the NHS. Indeed, you may feel that a person specification is superfluous. Despite that it may help at least to draw up a basic matrix (Figure 4.2).

There are, of course, dangers in these typed specifications; firstly, you may get who you think you want rather than who

	Essential	Desirable
Qualifications		
Experience		
Skills		
Personal characteristics		

Figure 4.2 A basic matrix for a person specification.

you need, and secondly, you can become hostage to a team that has deliberately arranged a specification that excludes all but its preferred candidate. Whatever the specification, it is important that the advertisement should not be too closely drawn and that the widest potential field of candidates is attracted.

Obtaining a shortlist

Before you advertise the post (it must be advertised) ensure that the following have been determined:

- a closing date
- an interview date
- a list of those proposed to sit on the interviewing committee
- an agreed job plan for the appointee.

For consultant appointments, the roles of those who will be on the interview panel and indeed involved in much of the remainder of the process, is carefully controlled by regulations. Shortlisting is carried out by the members of the Advisory Appointments Committee (AAC) and interviewing is also, in theory, conducted exclusively by the AAC. You should be familiar with the regulations that control these processes. They are explicitly and readably set out in *The National Health Service (Appointment of Consultants) Regulations 1996. Good Practice Guidance.* As new arrangements came into force on 1 April 1996, this guidance supersedes previous publications.

The AAC now consists of five core members. These will include: one lay member, who usually chairs the committee; the chief executive or his deputy; the medical director or his deputy; a consultant, normally from the relevant speciality and from the employing body; and lastly, a college-appointed assessor. The committee is required to have a majority of professional members and a majority of local members. University representatives will no longer be part of an AAC, except where the appointment is to a post which involves either substantial teaching or research commitments, or both. If more than one trust or hospital is involved it is allowed to have extra members from the other organisation.

The local team and potential colleagues will have views about the candidates and will wish to arrange the right appointment. Those representing the hospital on an AAC may have a difficult path to tread, in that they need to explore the views of the potential colleagues, even to the extent of having formal meetings with them to discuss CVs; but all must understand that no one can bind AAC members to a particular choice in advance. Candidates should be allowed an opportunity to visit the hospital and meet potential colleagues; there may even be a joint meeting with consultants and other candidates that they may attend. However, there is no obligation to attend such preinterview arrangements or "trials by cocktail party". Such gatherings are contentious and may be best avoided when planning appointments procedures. If there are such meetings care must be taken that questions are not asked of candidates that would not be allowed in a formal interview. In addition, be wary about unvalidated prejudice that may obtain through verbal references.

The dangers of unfairness in selection are manifold. Yet in our desire to be fair, give equal opportunities, and be politically correct, we run the risk of blunting our powers to choose the right candidate. Sticklers for correctness have suggested, for example, that preinterview visits to the hospital should be forbidden and that all candidates must be asked the same questions at interview. Fortunately, AAC guidelines do not require that and allow us, for example, to ask "questions to ensure that candidates, men and women, married or single, can meet the requirements of the job, for example where it involves unsocial hours". Even so, our means of selection are, to commercial organisations or hospitals in other countries, laughably rigid and inadequate. We do not test whether people might be able to work together, there is no psychological or specific aptitude testing or head hunting for elective appointments. The use of variations in salary to procure the best candidate is almost unknown. Too much is left to the single, highly structured meeting of a single committee, often filled with people who have minimal experience of the field to which the appointment is being made. Such committees run the risk of appointing the glib, the personable, and the paper-qualified candidate because of the shallowness of the assessment process.

References are largely worthless. They can confirm facts for the personnel department and check on absence records, but because of the dangers of litigation, few people are prepared to pass adverse comment, however honest. However, one must remember that a failure to comment on known poor performance in a candidate risks the individual being brought before the GMC for professional misconduct. What is sometimes informative, if unintentionally so, is to see who the candidate has *not* cited for references; if it is the candidate's most recent boss, one needs to wonder why.

The role of college representatives is somewhat misunderstood. They are there to ensure that candidates are appropriately qualified, not to appoint the oldest, longest serving trainee on the rotation into the post.

It is interesting that, although members of an AAC are supposed to have equal opportunities training and be fluent in interviewing techniques, they have only rarely had any formal training to ensure in particular that:

- all candidates are allowed equal time to talk
- questions are "open"
- each candidate is listened to for an equal length of time
- the interview time for each candidate is the same.

Trained interviewers can achieve a 1:4 interviewer to interviewee talk time ratio, whereas untrained interviewers' average ratio is 1:2, and for lay chairs 1:1.[10]

A source of guidance on interviewing is the BMA's *Guidelines for Good Practice in the Recruitment and Selection of Doctors*.

The appointment

When the AAC has made its recommendation, it is important to remember that it is just that. Indeed, an AAC may make more than one recommendation. The actual appointment is made by the "employing authority", for example the board of the trust, although there would normally have to be exceptional reasons why an appointment was not confirmed and it happens only rarely. If members of the team within the hospital feel that the AAC has forced an inappropriate consultant upon them, they do at least have one last opportunity to make an appeal before ratification of the appointment. The employing authority can authorise one of its members, for example the chief executive or the medical director, to approve the appointment at the time of the AAC, but they can only do so if the recommendation of the AAC is unanimous.

Induction

All staff joining a hospital should have a formal induction course, yet an Audit Commission assessment of trainees' hospitals showed that only 60% of all grades attend a general induction course for the hospital and only 30% attend one for their own speciality. For registrars these figures fall to 30% for a general course and 18% for a specific course. This is not the place to lay down the details of induction courses, but as a medical manager it is your responsibility to ensure that induction courses are in place and that the appropriate written material is available. A logical way to go about structuring an induction programme is to ask trainees who are leaving to say what it was they wished they had been told. In the absence of specific suggestions, proposed topics to cover on day one of induction programmes should include the following.

- Service processes and procedure (ordering investigations, hospital forms and notes, service departments, admitting and transferring procedures, discharge drugs, and procedures).
- Understanding hospital services (bleeps, switchboard, car parking, ID, support staff).
- Personal requirements (accommodation, housekeeping, catering facilities).

- Orientation to the new environment (mess and hospital facilities, meetings, timetables, rota).
- Essential practical skills (CPR, hospital computer, major disaster plan).
- Professional and financial concerns (P45, contracts, indemnity, rules relating to continuity of care, notification to coroner, liaison with GPs, etc).
- Educational arrangements (identification of supervisor and tutor, sources of career advice, details of study leave).
- Specific details of protocols and care pathways for patients of the team with which they will be working.

That is a lot to cover in one day but it is possible, although a lot of young doctors complain of being completely punch drunk at the end of their induction day and of having remembered almost nothing! A newly appointed house officer is likely to be frightened and apprehensive, emotions not conducive to detailed learning!

4.3 Managing conflict

Hospitals are stressed and stressful places by the very nature of what they do. Staff feel passionately about issues and have difficulty responding to change, to restrictions, and to the underprovision of resources. Difficulty is made worse at a local level by the size and undemocratic structure of the NHS as a whole, which throws up a lot of "us against them" areas of conflict. Sadly, there are also too many "us against us" issues concerning dominance, territory, and power; the same sort of issues you would see in a colony of apes. Most NHS consultants have tasted battle too many times in these areas to be naive or easily outflanked. But these conflicts are the stuff of management.

Doctors involved in management are uniquely placed to manage conflicts within the organisation because their privilege is to hold formal power through their office as managers at the same time as having credibility as clinicians. Furthermore, they can gain access to medical networks, can understand the clinical details of priorities, and crucially, can recognise clinical bluffing.

Donaldson[11] summarised the sources of power in an organisation as:

- holding formal authority
- controlling scarce resources
- having information
- possessing special expertise
- displaying the ability to cope with uncertainty
- commanding strong networks
- belonging to the dominant culture.

Medical managers qualify in almost all these categories. However, this does not guarantee ease in reducing conflicts, but the following suggestions may be useful.

- *Be impartial*: if this is made impossible by your position, be ready to use an outside arbiter to validate facts presented by both sides in the conflict and confirm the options that are available for resolving it. Management consultants are often simply making money out of their independence rather than any special skill or knowledge of the problem.
- *Avoid win/lose situations.*
- *Keep the temperature down*: but ensure that all protagonists are informed of the facts of the issues. It is more difficult to retain a partisan position when the larger picture has been spelled out clearly.
- Sometimes it is necessary to *marginalise one or more parties* in a conflict: this should not be done in an aggressive sense but softly, by exclusion from power areas or decision-taking bodies, whilst leaving bridges open. This is not Machiavellian, it is simply pragmatic.
- *Avoid trade-offs*: although some bargaining is inevitable in a negotiated solution to a conflict, try to avoid "buying-off" conflict if you can. Do not make promises of future benefits that you may not be able to deliver, or worse, which your successor will be expected to provide.
- *Involve other members of the team*: in the decisions that resolve the conflict.
- *Get the facts right*: disputes often focus on a disagreement about facts—try to get the correct information from an independent source.

Special areas of conflict

Dysfunctional teams

Few teams work well and a bit of dysfunction can add colour to the day; heaven preserve us from the endlessly sweet and helpful people who inhabited the books of our childhood, "Janet and John go to Genito-urinary Outpatients". The dysfunctional team to beware is the one that causes problems for patients and persisting unhappiness for the team members themselves; sadly, such teams are common and sorting them out is the clinical director's job.

The symptoms are fairly clear; personality clashes or individual failings are leading to measurable deficits in team performance, tears, complaints, letters, and the people who can leave are doing so. The ripples of disturbance spread outwards a long way from the primary protagonists. So what do you do?

Firstly, be honest. Was the team dysfunctional before you arrived or only since you arrived! If the latter then what has caused the problem. Is it (heaven forbid) because you have disrupted the status quo, changed rotas, failed to consult, made some bad appointments, pushed people into intolerable positions, or simply asked too much of the team? No! Right then, is it just a few difficult relationships or difficult people? Are these fixed personality traits or simply behavioural or performance anomalies only occurring in the context of this team? The latter may respond to some persuasion and open debate about the problem or one to one meetings to decide what changes may be made to resolve the conflict. In contrast, incompatible personalities in the team are a much more difficult problem to resolve and indeed if this is at the root of the problem it may not be soluble. There are many different personality types that can precipitate dysfunction in a team: one study collected 50 different ones—naggers and nitpickers, the scatterbrained, and the secretive; procrastinators and the pigheaded; whingers and workaholics are all there.[12] But what to do with them? My own view, based on observing attempts to resolve problems in teams, is that when difficult personalities perform dysfunctionally and upset patients in a clear and documentable way or fail to perform their defined tasks appropriately a straightforward disciplinary approach should not be shirked. Shirking diminishes your credibility with the team and may worsen the problem. Personality clashes that lead to an unhappy team, that nevertheless works adequately, need more careful handling. People with an established personality dysfunction are difficult or impossible to change and it is better to rearrange the team to avoid friction rather than try to rearrange the brains of the protagonists. That said, if it is really bad you may need to persuade one or more of the difficult ones to move or even leave—if you can; but tiptoe up to this solution carefully having consulted your director of personnel first.

I know of one trust which employed a psychologist to sit down with the dysfunctional team for a regular meeting to try to get them to love and honour one another: it did not work. The public airing of grievances exacerbated rather than ameliorated them. Murder was not committed in the meetings but it might have been! The outcome was that implicit dislike became explicit hostile disagreement. Poking a stick into a wasps' nest is a risky business. I appreciate that advising rearrangement rather than therapy is a cowardly if pragmatic way of addressing dysfunctional teams and I appreciate that communication is currently more fashionable than circumvention so do not let me discourage you from trying it. In doing so you might find *People Skills*, by Robert Bolton, helpful.[13]

Management versus the medical advisory committee

As a paid up medical manager your relationship with the medical advisory committee in your hospital may be fraught. The medical advisory committee, or whatever it is called in your hospital, is not just a parliament of consultants getting together disinterestedly to advise the management, it is, by contrast, the historical rump of the old consensus management process of the 1970s and 1980s and still expects to have power. Insofar as the membership contains the consultants the medical advisory committee still has great power and no manager should forget it, but it also has potential for great harm if allowed to fall prey to some of the archaic reflexes that such bodies can exhibit. The medical advisory committee may be like the Freudian "Id", the dreaming subconscious, the expression of inappropriate, infantile wishes in a disorganised way that can seem meaningful to itself though not to others; or, if you prefer a different psychological allusion, it may tend to display irrational Dionysian thought rather than rational Apollonian thought. Whether or not medical advisory committees are constructive and helpful is, of course, in their own hands. However bizarre their behaviour may seem, the management side should never ignore it and should make every effort to ensure that the medical advisory committee is well informed, ideally in writing and in advance, about what the organisation is doing, including facts on which decisions made the management side of the organisation are based (in particular, financial data). There are arguments about whether a medical advisory committee should be chaired by someone who is party to the current management and board thinking, for this may be valuable for resolving conflicts. One hopes that as more and more doctors have experience of the management of health care, polarisation between management and medical advisory committee will become less of an issue.

Purchasers of health care

For hospital trusts the relationship between medical managers and the purchasing authority and the public health doctors who work for or with them occurs at the collision point between one group within the NHS, the providers, who tend to feel that they should define what services are needed and how those services should be organised, and another increasingly empowered group, the purchasers, who feel it is they who better understand what is needed and are the proper definers of how it is to be delivered. So it is hardly surprising that sparks sometimes fly in meetings (politely of course). The competitive, market-based reforms of the Thatcher era and the recent splitting of purchasing from providing made many purchasers overbold in their dealings with providers. The public health doctors employed by purchasing authorities, and newly empowered by that, do not always realise the weakness of their data and the wider ramifications of flexing their purchasing muscles. In contrast, the medical and service directors of hospitals are frequently unsympathetic to the need for service rationalisation and the restrictions of an inadequate purchasing budget. As the participants, and the data on which decisions are made, become more sophisticated one hopes that cooperation will be more evident, though no doubt practising clinicians will forever be suspicious of the views of those who are not actually engaged at the coalface. Whatever the context, medical managers need to be aware of the potentially prickly nature of the relationship, particularly as the new primary care trusts start to flex their muscles.

4.4 Contracts and job descriptions

Older doctors consider medicine to be a vocation as well as a profession, and thus it might be considered in need of only the most minimal of contracts and a job description in the form simply of an indicative timetable of fixed commitments. My consultant contract when I was appointed was an all-embracing six paragraph statement simply reminding me of my responsibility to work to the best of my abilities for the hospital and its patients. The policing of such contracts was left to the conscience, peer pressure, and the General Medical Council (GMC). Unfortunately, there is a need to control the minority who abuse the spirit of such contracts and such contracts were, in addition, the product of a steady state and of no use to the manager afloat on a sea of continuous change. A disadvantage of the habit of bureaucratisation in the NHS, which itself reflects increasingly complex employment law, is that contracts have become more verbose, more detailed, and less flexible. Contracts between doctors and their employers are now underpinned by a job plan which defines the sessions that they are expected to work. The contracts themselves are primarily directive, identifying doctors' responsibilities, but they also carry some reference to the facilities that the employer will provide for doctors and the teams with which they will work. Additionally, they outline the framework which governs both parties' options when a change in job plan is needed.

As a manager—medical or otherwise—it is difficult to see how the work of doctors may be monitored or changed without such a template against which to measure it, but the risks of the plan itself and a managerial obsession with it are legion. The primary problem is that the very explicitness of a job plan may be perceived as implicitly denying trust and loyalty. Nevertheless, though there was much resistance to job plans when first proposed they are now generally accepted and understood not as a weapon of coercion but as a map of what doctors do and a starting point for planning a clinical service or for altering it. Their existence also allows a process of regular review.

The British Medical Association (BMA) issues guidelines on the completion of job plans which are sensible and do not deny the need for them. It is thus a rash medical manager who tries to impose some new format of their own and most do not, although it is reasonable to build on the concept of accountability which the job plan implies and to add other features. Your own organisation will have its habits in this respect, but as an example Guy's and St Thomas' Trust requires its consultants not only to complete a job plan but also to send in a diary of leave and study leave, and to account for how "flexible" sessions are being used. All this forms the basis for an annual appraisal.

The "new contract"

This second edition of *The Medical Manager* was cunningly planned to appear on the bookshelves at the same time as clinical managers were grappling with the implementation of a new consultant contract, but that will not happen for as we now know the contract was rejected in England and Wales, although accepted in Scotland. So what might have been an extended homily on the practical problems associated with its implementation has been shortened. Firstly, though, it is worth reflecting on the rejection itself. If you look at the outline contract that the BMA negotiated with the Department of Health (DoH) there is really nothing very draconian in it. In the frenzy of rejection there were claims that as soon as it was implemented managers would be forcing clinicians to work evenings and Saturday mornings for no extra pay, and the government was reminded of its commitment to "family friendly" employment policies. In reality, managers would have gained very little power in addition to what they currently possess. What the whole sorry business confirmed is that on the doctors' side there is still a deep mistrust of managers (many of whom are now doctors) and on the DoH side there still exists a robustly class-ridden view that consultants spend most of their NHS hours playing golf and doing private practice. After a period in which all parties, the Secretary of State, the DoH, the BMA, and the doctors, retreated to lick their wounds the Secretary of State confirmed that there would be no prospect of renegotiation of the contract and that piecemeal local arrangements would be encouraged so that the objectives of the new contract could be achieved. Conspiracy theorists might reasonably argue that that was his intention all along because it excludes the BMA from the process and it fits with his concepts of devolving some powers to trusts, which would not be so easy in the face of a continuation of a nationwide contract. The Secretary of State outlined his revised proposals in a document issued in January 2003, entitled *Improving Rewards for NHS Consultants*. The proposals are a complex mix of carrots and sticks for primary care trusts and trusts as well as for consultants. The carrots for consultants are the potential for non-recurrent annual bonuses for improved performance (though not in the form of premium rates for extra activity). The sticks include a threat that only good performers get access to discretionary points and clinical excellence awards, and that the rules relating to job plans, performance monitoring, and private practice will all be tightened up. Of course, once all that has happened consultants may feel more charitably inclined toward the "new" contract and the proposals note that where there is a "high level of consultant support for implementing the new contract" the contract may be implemented locally by trusts. "High level" is not defined, which is unfortunate and potentially dangerous. The covering letter notes that the views of SpRs will need to be taken into account but this requirement has mysteriously disappeared from the definitive document. All this represents a potentially nightmarish situation for clinical directors as they concurrently try to measure their teams' attitude to the proposals, decide what improved performance is needed and how to assess its achievement or non-achievement, and then decide if clinicians' input should propel them towards a clinical excellence award or whether they were entirely blameless in a failure to achieve what was—as is often the case—caused by some organisational or third party failure. How are clinical directors to respond to clinicians who take on national roles as examiners, editors, or assessors when current guidance no longer values these for clinical excellence awards and yet they detract from team productivity? There are no easy answers to this because as ever local freedoms will be restrained and monitored by central interference. All I can suggest is that you read the document and its successors carefully, try to work out what is between the lines as well as on them, and get together with your colleagues and the executive team in your own trust to put together a robust and simple system that will seem fair to your own teams, avoid missing out on the funds which are available for this, and try not to let this exercise further depress morale.

4.5 Appraisal and revalidation

Annual appraisal

The bureaucracy of management has an annual cycle to it: the financial year for setting and closing budgets; the medical staffing year revolving around the times of appointments for new staff; the business planning cycle rotating around what purchasers demand; and lastly, if you are a clinical director, you will need to fit into the cycle an annual review of job plans, incorporating an annual appraisal. You should review all staff. Managers (including you) are reviewed against the tasks that were set for them, trainee doctors against their educational targets, and consultants against their job plans. The process underpinning the annual appraisal of consultants will be familiar to you if you are a consultant; if it is not you can find it briefly summarised at http://www.doh.gov.uk/ nhsexec/consultantappraisal.

Consultant appraisal

It is part of the habit of the autonomy that British consultants enjoy that they may experience emotional difficulty in coming to terms with the notion of an annual appraisal. Therefore, from the outset you need to ensure that it is clear that appraisal is a two-way event, occurring in an informal setting, where you can both review the continuing appropriateness of the job plan, discover whether there are any skills that need sharpening, and what the organisation can do to assist in this process. Unfortunately, most clinical directors have no access to a budget for study leave and professional development with which to back up the conclusions of the appraisal, but at the very least the opportunity to review each consultant's contribution may help with the business planning process that follows it. Rightly or wrongly, annual appraisals seem rarely to be followed by significant change, but given the vagaries of the assessment process this may be sensible. Microsoft is said to grade its employees with marks one to five; four means exceptional, one means you are out! The other fashionable review process is the 360° review where each employee is assessed by their superiors, their peers, and their subordinates. It has been tried in the NHS as a pilot and seems useful if cumbersome, but the GMC is toying with the notion of using this technique as part of the appraisal needed for revalidation.

Any appraisal that reviews personal qualities rather than making an objective assessment of practical performance, adherence to job plan, etc, is a more risky activity. If it is to be done, of course, it must be conducted very, very sensitively and by someone competent enough and senior enough to undertake the exercise; I must, however, confess to sympathy with the view of Courtis:

> Staff appraisal is becoming more popular. Avoid it like the plague ... Good people take their merits for granted and sometimes don't want to know about their demerits. Average people can be demotivated by being reminded how average they are. Below average people can be hopelessly damaged by being told about faults which they do not have the brains or personality to surmount.[14]

Those truths apart there are other pitfalls in the appraisal process with which medical managers need to be familiar:[15]

- prejudice
- insufficient knowledge of the individual
- the "halo" effect of general likeability or recent events
- the difficulty in distinguishing individuals' performance from the context in which they work
- different perceptions of the standards required
- avoiding a difficult decision; everyone passes, no honours, no fails
- ignoring the outcome of the appraisal.

Many trusts now run courses for appraisers to make them more effective and all clinical directors ought to attend one, particularly as the momentum of the GMC revalidation process increases and the penalties for failed appraisal become more draconian.

A brief practical guide to appraisal may be found in *Medical Appraisal, Selection and Revalidation* by Gatrell and White.[16]

Appraisal processes should spend much more time focusing on facts, but the important facts about a single consultant's performance are usually unobtainable either because the right clinical data are simply not collected or because the data relate to the team not the individual. This is bound to change as better data are collected. An example is shown in Figure 4.3, which is a composite derived from one individual's audit data supplied to a specialist association's database. Importantly, it shows how the individual performs nationally relative to his or her peers.

Revalidation or reaccreditation by the GMC

At the time of writing the details of the GMCs plans for revalidating all doctors on a five-yearly cycle have not been finalised, but revalidation will certainly happen. The intention is to use consultants' annual appraisal forms and folders, and to have them assessed by GMC panels thus allowing "a seamless process which avoids complexity and duplication". That will, of course, depend on the quality of appraisal and its appropriateness as a vehicle for assessing whether doctors' performance is adequate across the whole range of performance and personal behaviour issues identified in the GMC's *Good Medical Practice*. Pilot studies are already suggesting that standard hospital appraisal folders will need to be backed up by some sort of professional colleague survey and patient questionnaire. The GMC is currently looking at more intrusive ways of appraising clinicians' health and their probity, but may fall foul of human rights legislation if it becomes too intrusive—especially in relation to health issues. Clinical directors need to keep a close eye on the revalidation debate lest they saddle their consultant colleagues with an annual appraisal process that is insufficiently thorough to allow subsequent revalidation. http://www.revalidationuk.

Draft summary report by consultant

*This report contains information on the
four index procedures for a consultant in
the period 1 Jan 1999–31 Dec 2001.
Negative outcomes were defined as
Died in theatre or Died in hospital*

	Carotid	IIB	Ruptured AAA	Unruptured AAA
Count	39	28	16	27
Observed mortality rate	0·00	14·29	6·25	7·41
SMR	0·00	1·01	0·14	1·65

**Observed and predicted mortality rates by procedure according
to the procedure-specific Bayes models**

Ruptured AAA

Recorded number of deaths = 1 out of a total of 16
Observed rate = 6·25% (95% CI: 0·33–32·29%) versus Predicted rate = 44·14% (95%
CI: 40·22–48·14%)
SMR = 0·14 (95% CI: 0·00–0·79)

Unruptured AAA

Recorded number of deaths = 2 out of a total of 27
Observed rate = 7·41% (95% CI: 1·29–25·75%) versus Predicted rate = 4·49% (95%
CI: 3·06–6·51%)
SMR = 1·65 (95% CI: 0·19–5·95)

Carotid

Recorded number of deaths = 0 out of a total of 39
Observed rate = 0·00% (95% CI: 0·00–7·39%) versus Predicted rate = 0·86% (95%
CI: 0·41–1·42%)
SMR = 0·00 (95% CI: 0·00–10·89)

IIB

Recorded number of deaths = 4 out of a total of 28
Observed rate = 14·29% (95% CI: 4·68–33·56%) versus Predicted rate = 14·18% (95%
CI: 10·74–15·83%)
SMR = 1·01 (95% CI: 0·27–2·58)

Figure 4.3 Draft of the type of annual summary report proposed by the
Vascular Surgical Society of Great Britain and Ireland (VSSGBI). It is
derived from one surgeon's audit returns and shows how he or she has
performed in relation to their peers as well as giving an indication of
how many index procedures he or she has performed and their death
rates. (Reproduced with kind permission of the VSSGBI.)

info is a useful and concise website with which to keep up to date. Information is also available at http://www.nhs.appraisals. nhs.uk and http://www.appraisaluk.info.

Appraisal of registrars

The appraisal of registrars in training rotations leading up to award of a Certificate of Completion of Specialist Training (CCST) is closely prescribed and monitored by regional training committees. Clinical directors are sometimes nonplussed to find the tutor in their directorate talking earnestly and at length about someone called "Rita" and may be too embarrassed to ask what they mean. In fact, the tutors are referring to a sequence of certificates that registrars in training may acquire if they are to be accredited, the Record of In-Training Assessment (RITA). RITAs are labelled from A to G and trainees only need records A, C, and G if all is going according to plan. C is the record the supervising consultant completes to confirm that all went well in the year, whereas RITA E assessment means trainees need to repeat that year. In summary, RITAs are as follows.

- RITA A *core information*: this must be completed at the outset of training and is used once only.
- RITA B *records changes in core information*.
- RITA C the *standard annual record of satisfactory progress*.
- RITA D completed if the *trainer recommends additional targeted training*.
- RITA E an indication that the *trainers are worried about the trainee*: require either more closely supervised training or a year to be repeated.
- RITA F records *out-of-programme experience:* must be filled in when a trainee temporarily leaves a programme for research or overseas experience if the national training number is to be retained.
- RITA G the *final record of satisfactory progress* through the training programme.

4.6 Rewards

It is normal to assume that everybody needs reward if they are to function well and to be happy. There are a few joyless psychologists who say that, by contrast, reward demotivates or encourages jealousy and a sense of injustice. However, that thesis does not stand up scientifically[17] and realistically we manage in a reward-driven environment. In the NHS we have rewards but they comprise a strange mix. Doctors have a sophisticated and generous financial reward system in the form of good salaries, augmented by merit awards, and that is in addition to the gratification they get from their status. Managers win promotion, performance-related pay, or some equivalent; manual workers receive a whole range of archaic supplements to their pay and the nurses ... Well, sadly, nurses have nothing much except public approval. All of us have the reward of working with and for people in a cooperative and worthy venture. It is a measure of the value of that ultimate job satisfaction that, despite the erosion of the sense of belonging to an institution, despite the abuses of our time and patience by worsening bureaucracy, and despite the culture of complaint, most of us love what we do. Very little erodes the four prime rewards of being a professional—collegiality, respect, variety, responsibility.

Nevertheless, as medical managers we should not expect these rewards to be the sole drivers of the workforce and we have an obligation to keep a regular eye on the rewards that staff receive, how they are given, and how best to build on them, or at worst, how to prevent their erosion. As a medical manager you need to understand the detailed mechanics of the finance reward systems that exist for doctors—discretionary awards and distinction awards.

Non-financial rewards

The capacity to reap the intrinsic rewards flowing from the exercise of compassion and the pleasure of doing a job well is something people bring with them to a job. It may be the greatest motivator of all and it is certainly the one cited by applicants for admission to medical school. It is not in the gift of managers, but other non-financial rewards are, importantly:

- setting identifiable and achievable goals, that is, feeling in control
- feedback to recognise achievement, that is, feeling valued

- allocation of responsibility appropriate to a person so that they can use their abilities optimally
- facilitation of personal development and further education.

For some staff these things are already formalised. House officers, for example, have little booklets given to them on their first day, explaining what their goals are. There are forms at the back of the booklet to be filled in jointly with their trainers to ensure that they have met to discuss progress and to recognise achievement. Simple they may be, but for some reason, popular they are not. The reasons for ignoring these structured systems of goal setting are one suspects largely laziness on the part of both parties. For house officers, goal setting is a relatively straightforward task. For other staff it may be a more difficult business, requiring assessment not only of the tasks that they need to achieve but also of the "core competencies" needed to achieve them. If these assessments are to be linked to financial reward, we also need a process for recognising extra effort beyond the basic task. It is important to remember, however, that research finds that financial reward is considered to be a surprisingly unimportant part of the motivation for most staff.

Your options for rewarding non-clinical staff are more limited, and these individuals feel put upon or out of control more easily, so this is an area that needs watching carefully. Your ward clerks, medical secretaries, and outpatient receptionists are valuable so you need to have a feel for their needs and grievances, rather than just take them for granted as most of us do.

Financial rewards

In essence, the NHS works on a system of "pay spines" with increments. Newly appointed SpRs start at a particular salary and move up to the top. Extra hours are paid but no account is taken of their skills or the effort they put in. There are no extrinsic incentives to perform well, although they need to pass their exams to stay in the grade, be tolerably competent, courteous and hard working if they are to be given references to rise out of one pay spine and into the consultant one. For managerial staff there are no exams and no major progression up a spine except by promotion. However, managers may be rewarded by performance-related pay and, less commonly, by skill-based pay. The problem with both of these systems is in assessing achievement. In essence, performance-related pay is a system for defining goals prospectively and then retrospectively measuring employees' performance in achieving them. Performance-related pay may be used to define progress through incremental grades or as an end of year bonus measure.

For employers difficulties lie in setting the goals accurately and in the subsequent assessment, particularly when weighing achievement in adverse rather than favourable environments. For employees, the rewards on offer may not justify the frustrations of achieving them, as 3–5% of salary is the usual sort of range for performance-related pay, and most will not get the full sum. Although widespread, performance-related pay is a difficult area for medical managers to become involved in and perhaps best avoided.[18] A study of performance-related pay in the public services, undertaken by the London School of Economics, concluded that it sours relationships, undermines morale, and encourages favouritism.

More popular are targeted rewards, either for groups or individuals. For example, operating theatre staff may all receive a one-off, end-of-year bonus if throughput has increased, or staff may be given individual payments if they have taken no more than a defined time off sick.

Discretionary points and distinction awards

When the original distinction award system was in place, doctors could receive C, B, A, or A+ awards. These represented a pensionable salary uplift of 25%, 50%, 75%, or 100%, respectively. Originally, once awarded they were for the duration of doctors' employment; now they are reviewed every five years, although it is rare for them to be taken away.

The C award was replaced in 1996 by the discretionary points system.

Discretionary points

Discretionary points are awarded only after consultants have achieved the maximum on the consultant salary scale. "They are paid at the discretion of the employer (ie the trust or health authority) in the light of professional advice." There are five points in the scale. Associate specialists and those with part-time and with honorary contracts are also eligible. Any number of points may be awarded to a consultant at one time but after an award of points a consultant should not normally be considered until two years have elapsed. The total number of points which a trust can award to its eligible consultants should not exceed the sum of 0·25 per eligible consultant. Eligible consultants are those who have reached the top of the incremental scale and who do not hold a B, A, or A+ award.

The whole process is run locally and medical managers, especially the medical director, should be central to the process of awarding points. The business of awarding discretionary points and distinction awards is invariably criticised (by the have-nots), and the process used must therefore be very open and the criteria for the awards plainly spelled out. The criteria which have been identified by the NHS Executive are shown in Box 4.1.

It is up to the local management to decide how to make the assessment, but a graded list from clinical managers is essential. A system of voting by the whole body of clinicians has a tendency to recognise the gregarious and the well-socialised to the detriment of quiet laboratory workers. Discretionary points are an improvement on the all-or-none quality of C awards, as they allow a better spread of reward. It might be thought that the slow progress to full allocation of points would delay the chance of a B award, but B awards are given for slightly different criteria and it is not necessary to have a full set of discretionary points before being considered for a B award.

Distinction awards

The world rewards the appearance of merit more often than merit itself.

La Rochfoucauld

The distinction award scheme was revised in 1995 and the details of its mechanics change each year so you need to keep up to date. This can be done by checking the *Guide to Consultants' Distinction Awards Scheme*, issued each year by the Advisory Committee on Distinction Awards (ACDA), and available on its website (http://www.doh.gov.uk/acda). Several important features may be summarised here, however.

Box 4.1 Guidelines on criteria for consultants' discretionary points (NHS Executive)

The following principles should underpin the local implementation of the scheme.

1. Discretionary points are *not* seniority payments, nor automatic annual increments.
2. Consultants in all specialities and all types of post are equally eligible and should be treated as such.
3. To warrant payment of a discretionary point, consultants will be expected to demonstrate an above average contribution in respect of service to patients, teaching, research and the management and development of the service.
4. Progression at each step up the discretionary point scale will reflect the increasing quality and range of the contribution made by the consultant. To attain the maximum of the discretionary point scale consultants will be expected to have demonstrated an outstanding contribution to services.
5. The criteria for payment of discretionary points should allow for contributions made in the following areas to be taken into account.

   Professional excellence, including:
   –quality of clinical care of patients
   –service development
   –professional leadership
   –improvements in public health.
   Significant contribution towards the achievement of local NHS service priorities.
   Undertaking recognised significant heavy workload or responsibilities in pursuit of local NHS service goals.
   Contribution to professional and multidisciplinary team working.
   Research, innovation and improvement in the service.
   Clinical audit.
   Administrative or NHS management contributions.
   Teaching and training, including:
   –training of junior staff
   –involvement in undergraduate or postgraduate teaching
   –public education and health promotion
   –contribution to training of other staff.
   Wider contribution to the work of the NHS nationally.

6. The differing opportunities and normal expectations associated with consultants in different fields will need to be taken into account in assessing the level of performance required in individual cases. For example, there will be a different expectation in terms of the research content of many honorary

(Continued)

Box 4.1 *(Continued)*

contract holders compared with consultants whose duties result in limited opportunities for research work. There would similarly be a different expectation in terms of the management and services development contribution of a consultant in public health medicine or dental public health compared with more clinically based specialities.

7. The resources available to a consultant, including supporting staff and facilities, and any particular difficulties that he or she may have had to overcome, should also be taken into account in judging the service contribution expected and provided.

8. In deciding payments employing bodies should ensure that consultants are treated equally regardless of their colour, race, sex, religion, politics, marital status, sexual orientation, membership or non-membership of trade unions or associations, ethnic origin, age, or disability.

- There is a fixed number of awards—about 14% of consultants hold an award and by retirement 25% will hold an award.
- Part-time consultants are paid pro rata in relation to their sessional commitment.
- No awards are granted after the age of 62.
- Rewards are reviewed every five years or earlier if there are "misgivings" about the award holder.
- Those in full-time management posts are not eligible but their awards are protected and reapplied when they return to clinical practice.
- Consultants who are re-employed into a substantive post after retirement can continue to be paid their award but not if the re-employment is as a locum.
- Recommendations may be made by individual trusts, by professional bodies and by individuals.
- There is an appeal system.
- A list of those who hold awards is made public.

To receive a B or A award, clinicians would normally need to be nominated by their trusts. Nowadays, the management side of a trust has a considerable input, so clinicians who abandon their NHS trust for the sake of a high-profile life of national or international activities are less likely than they were to be rewarded. It was not always so. I am aware of one consultant awarded a very high award for national work, who at the same moment, narrowly avoided disciplinary procedures within the trust because of poor attendance at fixed commitments. Such awards were doubly galling for trusts when the trust itself was responsible for paying the extra salary for largely absent clinicians. Things are better now that the emphasis is on honest hard work within the NHS, with much less attention to elitist activities outside the trust. Additionally, the fraction of the salary which is the distinction award, is now paid centrally instead of being taken from the trust's normal budget. Those likely to be nominated for a distinction award need to show in their submission form (known as the CVQ) that they have achieved in four "domains":

- delivering a high quality service
- developing a high quality service
- managing a high quality service
- research, teaching, and training.

As with the award of discretionary points, it is crucial that your organisation has—and is seen to have—a clearly defined system through which CVQs are processed and a transparent process that the review group uses to grade the CVQs and guide decisions (ideally a mixture of a points system and citation).

Once the trust itself has decided on its nominees, a regional, and then a national committee will process them before the final decision is made. The process takes almost a year and is complex. There are many checks and balances within it and it is fairly immune from inappropriate nominations. This does not, however, prevent the ritual expressions of outrage appearing in the press each year when the awards are announced. Such outbursts were previously directed at the secrecy of the process, but more recently have focused on a presumption of racial discrimination, sex discrimination, or favouring certain specialities (for some curious reason nuclear medicine emerges best). This is good fodder for the purveyors of political correctness, and for any politician who would wish to see an end to a system of merit awards, but it is rarely noted that such apparent inequalities are more a comment on the role played in the NHS by women and racial minorities than they are of the awards process itself. If women and ethnic minorities do not write papers or books or chair committees, are not elected to the council for this or that, or become professors, that may be a fault of the NHS—but it is not the fault of the distinction award process or the means by which we measure merit. The Commission for Racial Equality has looked at the scheme and was unable to find evidence of discrimination at work within it.

It is probably safe to assume that the existence of a distinction award system is a significant driver of consultant commitment to achievement over and above what is inherent in their daily work. Other systems of reward have been proposed to replace it, such as targets and rewards for clinical teams, as distinct from individuals. These do point up the importance of efficient team working and the need for mechanisms to encourage that, but they overlook the crucial importance of motivation working at a personal level. They also forget that many of the tasks in the NHS, especially those recognised by merit awards, are not team activities but individual ones.[19]

In its frustration at the consultants rejection, in 2002, of the proposed new contract the government quickly saw that it could use the rewards process as a means to increase its control over the consultant workforce, so radical changes may be expected.

And in case you were wondering, as I suspect you were, whether medical management posts increase the chance of being awarded a merit award, the answer is "Yes". Clinicians in management are more likely than their peers to have a merit award, but whether that is related to their management activities is not always clear.

4.7 Problems with colleagues

One of the most intriguing effects of time spent in medical management is the exposure it gives you to the character of your colleagues. Not only colleagues in particular, but doctors in general. I found this unexpected, for I thought I knew my colleagues; indeed I did, but only as friends where they were friends or as professional colleagues whom I judged as professionals. Were they a good opinion? Were they nice to patients? Were they prompt and diligent when referred a patient? What was surprising was how poor a predictor these skills are of the different abilities doctors now need. For example, the ability to work in teams, particularly when they are not the boss (the jargon phrase, I believe, is "cooperating in flatter, non-hierarchical structures"). Also, their ability to manage change. In the face of change some of the nicest and best doctors expose themselves as the most abject reactionaries, blind to reason, and prone to prima donna tantrums and the wilful misuse of facts. I do not know what percentage of clinicians fall into this category, but one analysis of non-medical organisation noted that 10% were "eagles" (leaders), 80% "sheep" (passively led), and 10% "mules" (obstructivist). I think the mule quota is a low estimate for clinicians, though I hope we also have more eagles.

Problems with colleagues fall into four distinct categories.

1. *The difficult colleague*: clinically competent, fine with patients and staff but often intransigent and uncooperative with managers and any others who try to control them.
2. *The naughty or improper colleague*: clinically competent, but rude and offensive to colleagues and patients, or whose timekeeping is unsatisfactory. These may be frank breaches of the trust's disciplinary regulations or may fall short of disciplinary error.
3. *The incompetent and/or dangerous colleague*: this group is dealt with in this section.
4. *The sick colleague*: sick doctors are discussed in Section 4.8, "The sick doctor".

An attempt should always be made to resolve these matters locally either within the directorate or within the trust or practice. If local resolution or even assessment seems impossible or fails then the National Clinical Assessment Authority (NCAA) may need to be involved or, less commonly, a rapid response team from the doctor's college. Suspending a doctor is an option open to trusts but it is a very crude response to problems with doctors and should only be used when there is very clear evidence of potential harm to patients if the doctor remains in post; it is not a mechanism for disciplining doctors. If you cannot deal with the problem internally, substandard practice that you think may be correctable should be referred to the NCAA; poor practice and behaviour that might bring doctors' continued registration to practice into question should be referred to the GMC. Matters of this seriousness must be discussed with the chief executive or the medical director and are not concerns where clinical directors should ever act alone.

The difficult colleague

Difficult colleagues are numerically only a small part of the workforce, but they are a real problem because they consume an inordinate amount of medical managers' time and energy. Unfortunately, you do not have a formula for dealing with them as you do with the doctor who is incompetent or who breaks the rules. Furthermore, obstructive colleagues are the very ones who are least likely to accept your right as a medical manager to ask for changes in the way they practise, and they certainly will not have any sympathy for your occasional need to pass comment on the way they conduct their personal clinical practice. If they are rabble-rousers and busy letter writers they become more than a nuisance and frankly are often damaging. Management books and courses are replete with advice on how to deal with this sort of person in an organisation, the "squeaky wheel", but in any particular instance the advice, like so much in management books, differs little from common sense. These books and courses will also recount the psychological personality types and parade for you a gallery of quirky personalities that can cause trouble. These certainly raise a smile when you recognise among them the obdurate, obstructive individual who is causing you so much trouble, but they rarely tell you *how* to deal with them. You may, however, find the "transactional analysis" view of interpersonal relationships helpful.[20] This looks at the kind of interaction you may have with your difficult colleague. Each of you, in any particular contact, is acting either as a parent or a child or an adult. Transactions may be:

- *complementary*: natural relationships such as parent–child or adult–adult
- *crossed*: where the opening approach receives an inappropriate response, for example, manager: *"Can we discuss how we are*

going to deal with the waiting list?" (adult), clinician: *"No, I'm too busy and it's your problem not mine"* (child)

- *ulterior*: these are more complex but the most common is exemplified by the real message being disguised under an explicit socially acceptable message.

Transactional analysis stresses the importance of looking at the *feelings* that generate the heat in transactions that are seemingly about *facts*.

Of course, you should in the correct parental, adult way try to explain and persuade, but I have to conclude that to protect yourself and the other work that needs to be done, obdurate mules are often best managed simply by being marginalised, and the river of events merely allowed to flow on around them. There are, however, some basic principles to apply in your dealings with obdurate colleagues, namely.

- Listen courteously and open mindedly.
- Do not allow your replies to be aggressive or threatening. Somebody with a grievance is more of a problem than somebody who is simply a nuisance.
- Leave bridges open for late conversion.
- Do not become involved in protracted exchanges of letters.
- Make sure your policy is shared with your managerial colleagues to avoid the obdurate clinician simply trying to bypass you.
- Always refute quietly but publicly attempts to raise the temperature by the use of false data.
- Try to explain the broader picture. The obdurate clinician is usually more concerned about small and personal issues and has not, cannot, or will not see the broader picture.

In these matters most of one's colleagues are supportive and understand the issues, and therefore one should not let them down by taking the easy option of giving in to the noisy one.

The naughty or improper colleague

Doctors get away with a lot that they should not. Latitude in personal attendance and behaviour has often been tolerated out of an archaic subservience to an imagined professional ethos that protects and insulates them from the work-a-day world. Bad behaviour, such as rudeness, is often tolerated in doctors as a charming quirk of character—the "Sir Lancelot Spratt" phenomenon; charming quirks of character that when exhibited by a porter lead promptly to his/her dismissal.

The social culture in which we work has changed and although quirkiness itself may lend colour to a drab world, quirkiness that is naughtiness or impropriety needs to be changed. No one is better placed to do this than clinicians in management. Recurring problems that they will have to deal with are non-attendance and late attendance at fixed commitments, rudeness to patients and staff, and denigration or harassment of other staff. In my experience the difficulty in these situations is getting the problem into proportion and not over- or underreacting. Your non-involved colleagues will be watching very closely. The following suggestions may be useful.

- *Get the facts right*: if there is an allegation of rudeness or harassment elicit the facts from the victim in writing. People are often unwilling to do this, but without something solid to back you up you are unlikely to make much impact on the malefactor who simply denies it all. Victims may not be prepared to put it in writing but you do at least need to get a promise that they will speak about the issues in front of you with a witness present. If possible, it is wise to obtain corroboration. Is it just one person who finds the doctor difficult or offensive, or is it a shared perception among the team? Is the event about which the complaint is made merely an opportunity to convert a longstanding grudge into punitive action?
- Having decided to go ahead *deal with the matter firmly*: the first conversation need not be formal but subsequent ones should be.
- Remember that *any formal meeting to discuss a problem should be documented* (I send a letter afterwards summarising what was said): try to have a colleague manager with you and offer the clinician in question a chance to bring someone with them.
- *Always try for an informal resolution*: formal procedures are protracted, time consuming, painful, and sometimes

even counterproductive, and at the very least they are a distraction.

- Occasionally the clinician in question will agree that *help is needed to improve their attitude*, although this is rare: there are no equivalent of Maoist re-education camps available in the NHS; it is hoped that in future the NCAA will act as a network of trained, sympathetic clinicians and/or psychologists so that colleagues who want help may be referred outside the organisation for that help.
- Lastly, remember that *people who are causing problems may simply be markers of a dysfunctional team*: being made scapegoats or just not adequately supported.

In this section I have not outlined a sequence of formal disciplinary procedures. Although these tend to be much the same from trust to trust, they often differ in detail and it is important that medical managers read their own trusts' disciplinary procedures very carefully before instigating any formal disciplinary process. We are all familiar with the fictional policeman/woman who fails to achieve the true guilty verdict on a criminal simply because he/she neglected to act "by the book" or read the suspect his/her "rights". Formal hearings in the medical context should also be done by the book, so you ought to have read it! Do not expect the regulations about disciplinary proceedings to be easy reading, and in general it is advisable to consult your director of personnel about the practicalities before acting.

If you are in a position where a disciplinary process becomes necessary, the "Hot Stove" principle of Macgregor is a useful *aide-mémoire* to ensure your evenhandedness and consistency. Douglas Macgregor was an American industrial psychologist who likened the well-tailored disciplinary process to touching a red hot stove:[21]

- the burn is immediate, so there is no question of cause and effect
- there was a warning: the stove was red hot, and you knew what would happen if you touched it
- it is consistent: everyone who touches the stove gets burned
- it is impersonal: you get a burn not because of who you are but because of what you have done.

Political correctness issues

Formal complaints about staff behaving in a "politically incorrect" way seem rare, but they are potentially difficult to deal with. Doctors often behave in a "politically incorrect" but well-meaning way. The normal banter between male doctors and female nurses is long established but potentially misinterpretable in the current climate. Many doctors find the linguistic fascism of the new correctness both ludicrous and unhelpful, and this may make potential trouble for medical managers who may not understand the passion that some people attach to political correctness. An event which may seem to you to be absurdly trivial but which is perceived by someone on the staff as a major injustice may trip you up, and the humourlessness of the victim culture that underlies the political correctness movement may depress and irritate you. Nevertheless, mixed in with these irritations are true injustices that need acting upon.

The most common way in which political correctness issues arise are:

- as alleged harassment, usually racial or sexual
- as attempts to make you change language or procedures to be politically correct
- equal opportunities policies interacting with normal appointment, reward, and disciplinary activities.

The process for dealing with the first should be straightforward in that it should not differ from any other disciplinary process and your trust's disciplinary rules should explicitly include harassment. Difficulty arises where harassment is perceived but not intended—where politically incorrect speech, for instance, is perceived as harassment. This may afford you an opportunity for some difficult tightrope walking, particularly at present where many disciplinary procedures, themselves couched in politically correct language, state that harassment exists if a person believes themselves to be harassed.

The incompetent colleague

We know that doctors are not perfect and the clinical skills and human relations of many are suboptimal. We know that medicine deals at its core with the fallibility of humans and that doctors are no different from other humans, but nevertheless a small number are simply so bad as to be dangerous, though not as many as the media and the government would have the public believe. If the quality of medical care is to improve and if doctors are to be safer we need to have processes in place to identify and then improve or remove dangerous doctors and to improve the standards of safe but poorly performing doctors.

A sequence of milestones must be passed before these objectives may be achieved.

- *Insight*: doctors need sufficient insight to understand that they need continuous refreshing and re-education. This dimension is too often missing, although evidence suggests that the prevalence of audit meetings and the habit of peer group review is gradually eroding this misplaced confidence. Doctors also need insight into their own illnesses and their ways of dealing with their own illnesses, something they tend to do badly through an innate perception that "doctors don't get ill".[22]
- *Identification*: awareness that if others are repeatedly clinically risky then one does not just look away. All clinicians have a duty to protect patients. Doctors who are quick to point out the dangers of an underfunded NHS are sometimes slow to act to do anything about a fully funded but incompetent colleague.
- *Retraining*: once poor performers are identified, by themselves or others in a hospital setting, retraining options must be available if needed and support must be provided for aged or ailing doctors. If the problem is illness, whether psychiatric, drug induced, alcoholic, or whatever, support is needed for that too (*see* Section 4.8, "The sick doctor"). A more difficult situation is found when doctors fail to understand that they are performing badly, and reject advice. A more formal process is then needed to protect patients.
- *Professional review*: only if internal hospital processes fail or for some reason are impossible will the problem need to be passed to the NCAA or the General Medical Council (GMC). It should be noted that even if hospital internal

processes are underway or successfully completed, reports about malperforming doctors may reach the GMC by other routes, for example the public or whistleblowers. In relation to the NCAA and the GMC it is important to remember that poor performance is not about a single episode, it is about consistent or repeated failures, and it is about the performance of clinical tasks. It must never be a way of resolving internal trust wrangles about disciplinary matters such as late attendance.

When dealing with defects of performance, whether internally or by use of the NCAA or GMC, care must be taken to confirm that the defects are real and documentable. It is not sufficient for a cabal of doctors and managers to take against clinicians because they are inept, lazy, or not to their taste and then expect the GMC to resolve the problem for them.

The intention of the NCAA process is remedial not disciplinary. However, if the investigation reveals information which suggests that disciplinary procedures are needed by the trust then the GMC will trigger those processes.

For details of the NCAA and GMC professional review processes *see below*.

In all disciplinary and performance enquiries remember:

- get the facts right
- act promptly
- act openly
- keep records
- do not take sides
- take advice from the personnel department and the medical director
- remember the objective is the protection of patients.

"Shop-a-doc"

A lot of heat has been generated by the debate about doctors telling someone about colleagues who are performing poorly. The reflex not to "sneak" on a colleague to someone in authority is deep-rooted in the English psyche. EM Forster is famously quoted as saying he hoped he would have the courage to betray his country rather than a friend. The "shop-a-doc" fuss is more subtle. It arises from attempts following the 1995 Health Department report, *Maintaining Medical Excellence*, to enshrine in doctors' contracts an obligation to report poorly performing colleagues. Quite reasonably, the BMA and others objected to this, pointing out that it was an ethical not a contractual issue. One hopes that no one quibbles with the ethical principle. The GMC rules are quite explicit on this, and indeed in the folder that contains each doctor's annual registration certificate there is a list of duties for doctors, one of which clearly states "act quickly to protect patients from risk if you have good reason to believe that you or a colleague may not be fit to practise".

The issue then is that dangerous doctors need to be identified whatever your queasiness about the process. But how do we disentangle gossip from reality and protect patients while being fair to colleagues? The answer lies in a clear and accepted process. This is more likely to succeed if led by doctors, so they have the responsibility to establish, communicate, and police the policy. Traditionally, medical advisory committees like to do this separately from the hospital administration, and the process of the "three wise men" existed to deal with part of the problem in relation to sick doctors. Nevertheless, in the current situation where there are many doctors in management it is neither appropriate nor necessary for medical advisory committees to keep these issues "in-house"; clinical directors and/or the medical director must always be informed that a process is underway even if the medical advisory committee and its officers are to be the prime movers. There are those who object to this, but they should remember that a trust carries both legal and moral responsibilities for its patients as well as bearing the financial risks of medical negligence. If a group of clinicians takes upon itself the responsibility for deciding about inept colleagues and does so without the knowledge and cooperation of the trust, the members of the group put themselves personally in a difficult position if a disaster occurs.

Referral to the National Clinical Assessment Authority

The NCAA was set up in 2001, on the recommendation of the Chief Medical Officer, to provide a neutral body for helping NHS employers "deal in a more timely and consistent way with doctors whose performance gives cause for concern" in relation not just to clinical skills but interpersonal ones as well. The NCAA exists to support doctors and their employers and thereby indirectly the public. It does not take direct referrals from the public but does have a mechanism for responding to the concerns of whistleblowers. Although it deals with all grades of clinical staff, it expects that the normal performance review mechanisms already in place for trainees will be the preferred route for that group and therefore consultants, NCCGs, and locums will be its main clients. There will, of course, be some overlap between the work of the NCAA and the GMC and, to a lesser extent, CHAI, but the NCAA is quite distinct from those other bodies in that it acts only with the doctors or their employers to improve the performance of unsatisfactory doctors whilst they remain in post and it deals not with single events but problems that are "serious and repetitious" that with help are judged to be amenable to correction. The remit of the GMC is different. It exists to determine whether doctors' performance or behaviour is bad enough to require removal from the Medical Register. The interests of CHAI lies in the organisation as a whole and it is looking for departures from good clinical governance and for system failures.

NCAA procedures occur in three stages.

1. Giving advice and taking a referral.
2. Planning and undertaking a formal assessment.
3. Reporting back and action planning.

All this is paid for by the NCAA.

The NCAA aims to address all three possible causes of lack of "clinical capability": health problems, behavioural difficulties, and lack of clinical ability. It is anticipated that most cases will be dealt with at stage one, the advisory stage and that only 10% will progress to stages two and three. Such progression will only happen when the employer, the NCAA, and importantly, the doctor agree that it might be useful. The details of this process are clearly laid out in the NCAA website (http://www.ncaa.nhs.uk) and in its *Handbook*, but beware, at the time of writing there was a considerable backlog of cases and the NCAA was having difficulty recruiting assessors.

Sadly, on a few occasions all the in-house effort and outside support does not suffice and the GMC will need to become involved, or else all the options for support will have been bypassed by a complainant who goes straight to the GMC.

General Medical Council procedures

It is as well to remind ourselves of the background to these procedures by remembering that the GMC was created under a Medical Act of Parliament in 1858 specifically to improve medical education and to set standards of practice. It exists to protect the public interest and the good name of the profession. The GMC is made up of doctors elected by the profession, by university medical schools and postgraduate institutions, and lay people who are nominated by the Privy Council. In recent years the number and influence of the lay membership has increased. The GMC is an independent statutory body and is not a government agency, not part of the NHS, not involved in organising or providing health care, not an employer of the medical workforce in this country, nor is it the doctors' union. It's structure and function, as you will know, has been widely criticised by everyone—both lay and medical—and it is currently being reorganised.

Procedures for assessing performance come under the "Fitness to Practise Division", which was created in 1858 to deal with serious professional misconduct and convictions. In 1980 a further Act was passed through parliament to deal with health issues of doctors that were sufficiently serious to impair their fitness to practise. The performance procedures have been introduced to deal with *seriously* deficient performance. The GMC is not involved in dealing with variations of practice which do not threaten the patient or public.

Within the Fitness to Practise Division there is an organisation for screening all complaints received. The screeners are members of the GMC who are given specific training to make discreet enquiries to identify whether there is a *prima facie* case requiring further investigation. If the screener decides there is concern then health issues take precedence over conduct issues, over performance issues.

The health procedures are private and confidential, and aim to be remedial. If doctors cooperate the matter may be handled entirely locally and assessment is based on the opinion of medical experts.

Conduct procedures, on the other hand, are formal, public, and adversarial. They are designed to deal with specific incidents, but do not allow the GMC to investigate a doctor's general standard of practice. There are no provisions for formal counselling, retraining, or reassessment where there is evidence of poor performance. Therefore, conduct procedures may investigate particular serious incidents but cannot investigate patterns of poor performance.

Performance procedures have been introduced to fill this gap and have two main purposes: to protect the public and to give deficient doctors a chance to improve.

The mechanics by which the GMC validates complaints, investigates them and then maybe proceeds with formal hearings is complex and evolving, and it would not be useful to burden you with them here. We hope you will never need to know about them. However, if you do, you should know that the GMC issues booklets for complainants and for doctors about its processes and these are available on the GMC website (http://www.gmc-uk.org). Also available on the website (but not in booklet form) is information for clinical managers advising them when they should use their own procedures and when they should consider contacting the GMC about doctors' performance.

4.8 The sick doctor

Contrary to their expectations doctors get sick. We have already seen that they are stressed and as a consequence have a high incidence of psychological illness, drug-related problems, alcohol abuse, and suicide, quite apart from the normal gamut of physical illness. Ramirez and colleagues found a 27% prevalence of psychiatric morbidity in consultants.[23] Their higher risk of suicide has been documented at 1·1 to 5·7 times that of the normal population.[24] They have a three times greater incidence of cirrhosis than the general population.[25]

Doctors with physical disease have a familiar and inappropriate set of responses to that disease:

- denial
- failure to seek prompt advice
- using advice gleaned from colleagues in the corridor
- avoiding GPs and occupational health doctors
- self diagnosis and self medication
- are unwilling to take time off because of professional pressures and loyalty to colleagues. Doctors take only 1% of their time as sick leave compared with the NHS average of 5%,[26] and three-quarters of doctors admit to having worked when they felt so ill that their judgment was impaired.[27]

This is a very unhealthy situation. Nevertheless, consultants may use their experience and contacts to ameliorate the ill effects of this, but doctors in training do not have these options. Questionnaires and studies show unacceptable levels of physical and mental stress among doctors in training caused by the intensive workload and unfamiliar pressures of responsibility. Most of the calls received by the BMA Helpline are from doctors aged between 21 and 25.[28] There is little evidence that the trend to reduce working hours has helped in this; it has merely increased the stress during the reduced working hours.

"Burn-out" is not in a medical sense a disease, it is an outcome of chronic stress in the context of frontline clinical staff that may occur in anyone faced with high stress levels and inadequate resources with which to deal with the situation. It is often a prelude to frank physical illness and needs to be dealt with as a "sickness" issue. Managers need to be aware of the symptoms: exhaustion, cynicism, detachment from the job, a sense of ineffectiveness, and often deteriorating performance at work.

You may say that none of this is medical managers' responsibility because there are supposed to be different channels for helping with these problems. Medical managers, however, should not ignore health issues in staff who are their responsibility and that, of course, includes not only doctors but also nurses and others.

Medical managers must be involved because:

- they have pastoral responsibility for the employees in their ambit
- stress and illness, in particular psychological problems, drug, and alcohol abuse, may affect the effective care of patients, even their safety.

Their involvement, however, may be difficult as many employees, unfortunately, regard medical managers as Dickensian characters usually trying to screw more work out of them and poised to fire them if they have problems. One way around this is to ensure that the speciality tutor or some other non-managerial clinician takes responsibility for the day-to-day welfare of trainees. Similarly, there should be a specific, named person with pastoral responsibility for nurses and others. Occupational health arrangements should be clearly advertised and counselling available. Most doctors prefer to be counselled offsite and should be aware of the BMA Stress Helpline (tel: 08459 200169 or 0645 200169) which is open 24 hours a day and is also available for doctors' families. There is also the National Counselling Service for Sick Doctors (tel: 0870 241 0535; website: http://www.ncssd.org.uk) and The Sick Doctors' Trust (tel: 01252 345163; website: http://www.sick-doctors-trust. co.uk). In addition, the Association of Anaesthetists have a Sick Doctors' Scheme (tel: 020 7631 1650), there is a specific support group for those with drug problems (The British Doctors and Dentists' Group, tel: 0207 4867 4445) and for those with mental illness (The Doctors' Support Network, tel: 07071 223372; website: http://www.dsn.org.uk). These do not, of course, resolve the problem of doctors' unwillingness to admit to illness or to seek help. Cultural changes are necessary if this is ever to be resolved.

Doctors must take more responsibility for their peers and be prepared to discuss illness perceived in colleagues. In addition, the system as a whole needs to pay particular attention to confidentiality where staff illness is concerned. This will require, for example, ensuring that test results are not generally available on the hospital computer system. All this, however, leaves a hiatus where patients are concerned. Clinical directors or medical directors are responsible for ensuring that sick doctors do not present a threat to patients. In this there is no difference from their responsibilities in relation to incompetent doctors. The current mechanisms to deal with the dangers presented by sick doctors, however, are somewhat confused. If sick doctors have insight and present themselves to a GP or occupational health doctor, it is that clinician's responsibility to advise them that they are a risk to patients. However, if doctors fail to present, refuse advice, or have no insight into the problem, we must rely on colleagues or other staff to sound the alarm. In that event the "three wise men" procedure comes into effect. "Three wise men" is the slang term for "a subcommittee of the Special Professional Panel set up under HC82/13". Although this is an old health circular, it has not been cancelled, and anyone involved in the difficulties concerning the management of sick doctors should read it. (I would not normally advise reading health circulars as a pastime but this is an exception.) In summary, the health circular says:

[In paragraph 3] There should be a special professional panel set up by the medical executive committee consisting of members of the senior medical staff from which a small sub-committee should be appointed. The sub-committee should receive and take appropriate action on, any report of incapacity due to physical or mental disability including addiction. It does not have a duty to report back to the panel.

[In paragraph 6] Information will normally be given in the first instance to one of the members of the panel but sometimes to the chairman of a clinical division. It may come from a variety of sources and may relate to medical or dental staff of any grade. It will usually be given by a colleague but may be from another discipline or from a general medical or dental practitioner.

[In paragraph 8] The sub-committee should make such confidential enquiries as are necessary to verify the accuracy of any report. Whilst they are not required to establish positively that the possibility of harm to patients exists or to make a clinical diagnosis, nevertheless if they are satisfied the report has substance the practitioner should be told of its contents and be given the opportunity to be interviewed by the sub-committee ... If the sub-committee feel that the possibility of harm to patients cannot be excluded by the exercise of their influence ... they should bring the circumstances to the notice ... of the medical officer of the employing authority.

[In paragraph 9] It is the responsibility of the officer of the employing authority who receives the report from the sub-committee under this procedure to decide what further investigations are necessary. If it appears that a question arises that the doctor's fitness to practice may be seriously impaired ... consideration should be given as to whether the circumstances might justify report to the registrar of the General Medical Council for consideration in accordance with the procedures of the council's health committee.

This remains one of the few formal responsibilities still vested in the medical committee of the hospital rather than the medical director. However, insofar as members of the panel might be held legally responsible for any harm to patients caused by a clinician who was unfit to practise, and who had been notified to them, the problem has been glossed over; it seems prudent that the chairperson of the panel should maintain close liaison with the medical director. The "three wise men" procedure is best viewed as the first, informal stage of an assessment process which then progresses to the NCAA if a more formal process is needed.

It ought not to be necessary to say so, but experience suggests that it is important to remember that patients' welfare comes first, and that "buddy relationships" between clinicians which conceal incapacity are, in the long run, in nobody's interest.

We should not leave this subject without noting that most ill health in NHS workers is psychological and much of that is a consequence of unsatisfactory working environments, overwork, and poor organisation—all of which is in theory at least under the control of managers.

4.9 Professional and personal development

Professional development for clinicians generally

"Professional development" is a term attracting much lip service, although not always the commitment of a budget. As far as clinicians are concerned it is, at its simplest, continuous medical education (CME), the refreshing of old skills and knowledge, and the learning of new skills. It is an obligation inherent in the life of professionals, but if you see the annual returns detailing your colleague clinician's study leave you will probably be surprised at the range of uptake from the man who never misses a chance to fly away to meetings or slip off to his college (absences, which with other leave, not infrequently add up to more than three months of the year for academics) and contrast this with the overcommitted clinician who rarely misses a clinic and never takes study leave.

The obligation to arrange CME remains a professional and ethical issue in Europe and the format of CME has changed little over the years. Yet we have no proof that hours spent in these traditional forms of CME—journal clubs, postgraduate meetings, deaths and complications meetings, professional group conferences, etc—actually improve our performance as clinicians. One study found that the number of reported CME hours correlated positively with lower competence!, an association of course, rather than a cause.[29] If then medical managers are to put their hands to the oars to try and facilitate CME in their units, they need to remember that simply pressuring people into attending PGME meetings is not necessarily the correct answer. The cooperative and reflective medical team is itself an educational engine, but the crucial element is the efficiency of doctors' capacity for self-directed learning and that is not something that may be imposed. Actually, most doctors do not know what the phrase "self-directed learning" means or implies but do it unconsciously.

In spite of anxieties about the effectiveness of formal CME, its promulgation and measurement, though not of course its funding, continues to be a growth area in the NHS. In the USA, most speciality board certification is now limited to 7–10 years, with recertification necessary at the end of that time. This seemingly straightforward process has proved to be a financial and educational minefield and may not deliver any better results than other less formalised systems. Recertification in the UK looks set to be a more subtle process with the net cast wider to collect evidence of continuing competence. Whatever the pundits might say about the value of enforced CME, it remains an obligation on medical managers to work to ensure that adequate time and funding is made available for such leave.

Educating clinicians about management

Professional development for clinicians in the form of "management training" is heavily proselytised. Trainees doubt that they will get a consultant post without having been on a "management course". This is sad, as a badly run course, orientated towards business management seems often to raise antibodies to management in the very trainees who will be needed in the future to help manage the service. I have to express a bias here. I would personally prefer clearly to separate three types of management training.

- *NHS citizenship*: which is about how the NHS works.
- *Personal development*: which is about developing human skills which would be valuable in a management role but might currently be missing—communication, assertiveness, chairmanship, interviewing, that sort of thing. This is covered later in this section.
- *Management training*: which deals with the specific skills needed to run the health business—personnel, finance, contracting, etc.

All doctors need the first, most will need some of the second, and at some stage some may need the third, but certainly not at the undergraduate stage, as has been proposed.[30]

The important part is the NHS citizenship training and that should indeed begin at undergraduate level where it is often dressed up as a course in public health. It should improve awareness of the mechanisms of the NHS, its financial and organisational constraints, ethical issues about rationing, and a bit about practicalities such as equal opportunities. There is no reason why clinicians need go outside their own hospitals for this sort of training. It is probably more acceptable if it is merged with other educational activities within the hospital and it is medical managers' obligation to arrange such sessions and coax clinicians to attend. A series of such sessions in our trust, aimed primarily at younger clinicians, has been gratifyingly well attended and better received than conventional wisdom would predict.

For established clinicians, management training or professional development may usefully be tied to what they need to know; that is to say, a basic series of skills training should be made available (for example, non-discriminatory interviewing, staff assessment, communication skills) and targeted education aimed at improving his comprehension of changes in the NHS (such as process improvement, audit, EBM, the roles of CHAI, NICE, and all the other acronymic genies).

Professional development for medical managers

Although it is fairly clear what professional development means for clinicians, it is uncertain exactly what it means in the context of medical managers. One could say that it is simply something done by, to, or for medical managers to make them better managers, but better at what?

For medical managers such development can fall into one of two categories:

- moulding the person to the corporate objectives
- developing skills in the person to enable them better to fulfil their job.

Moulding the person to fit the corporate plan

Many of the so-called management training proposals for doctors and students within the NHS at present fall into this category. The idea is that if you show how the finances work, how the system works, what the constraints are, and how to function in teams; if you explain to them the mechanics of purchasing and the inevitability of rationing then they will accept it and work better, more comfortably, and quietly within the system. Whether that really is the outcome remains to be seen, but most hospital trainees now have some of this type of management training. Perhaps as a consequence some take a more understanding stance in relation to the running of the service but others do not and remain bitter recidivists. I doubt if it is known how many have been converted and, in view of the changing background against which such management development occurs, how can it be known? In the meantime, as an act of faith, we go on encouraging trainees and new consultants to go on management courses and perhaps, improperly, we provide the money for those courses with more readiness and enthusiasm than we do for their CME.

Developing the skills of medical managers

It is worth asking whether there actually exists a body of knowledge and skill that managers can learn and, indeed, does managerial competence exist as a measurable skill? It is an article of faith in the development business that such skills can be taught and learnt, just as it is an article of faith that certain core competencies are needed to fulfil the job.

Core competencies In their review of the management skills of clinical directors, Gatrell and White[31] listed the competencies (Box 4.2) and, commenting on their assessment of clinical directors in post based on 1400 questionnaire returns and 230 interviews, these authors noted that many clinical directors have met their own needs through experiencing problems and seeking answers and information themselves, but that "there are many who have learned to get by with a mixture of common sense, avoidance, information

---

Box 4.2 Competencies required for a clinical director

- Implementing patient satisfaction indicators
- Negotiating contracts
- Monitoring business performance
- Business planning
- Managing a budget
- Generating income
- Handling official complaints
- Managing organisational crisis
- Using management information systems
- Problem solving and decision making
- Counselling colleagues and subordinates
- Chairing meetings
- Negotiating
- Conducting appraisal interviews
- Conducting selection interviews
- Delegating work to colleagues
- Acting as a figurehead
- Understanding and influencing organisational culture
- Managing professional reputation in the context of managerial work
- Implementing difficult non-clinical decisions
- Adopting an ethical management stance
- Handling uncertainty

(Reproduced from: Gatrell J, White T. *Medical Student to Medical Director—a development strategy.* NHS Training Division, 1995.)

Box 4.3 Competencies required for a medical director

- Recruitment, selection of non-medical staff
- Pursuing equal opportunities
- Developing terms and conditions of employment
- Non-clinical staff training
- Staff appraisal
- Implementing decisions
- Disciplinary procedures
- Implementing patient satisfaction indicators
- Dealing with the media
- Negotiating
- Conducting interviews for grievance and discipline

(Reproduced from: Gatrell J, White T. *Medical Student to Medical Director—a development strategy*. NHS Training Division, 1995.)

---

from peers and bluff". In addition to listing the skills required of a clinical director, they also listed those required for a medical director (Box 4.3). The difficult issue is how to decide which of the skills listed can and should be taught formally. Many are extensions of the skills already learnt as a doctor. One needs to ask whether some of the competencies defined as desirable are really appropriate skills for a doctor-manager to learn, or whether their presence on the list is merely a reflection of an inappropriately defined job. Although in their report Gatrell and White indicate that the respondents to their questionnaires *asked* for training and development, I am not aware of any study that shows improved performance as a result of such formal management training. Lik Mui[32] looked at organisational problems experienced by medical directors and found that with time in post medical directors became better at the tasks, regardless of whether or not they had had training. When he looked at personal problems (Box 4.4) he found less improvement with time.

One interpretation of the list of areas that medical directors found difficult is that their jobs as defined are too broad, their timetables too full. It is probably the job that should be altered in these circumstances, but if it is not then perhaps there is some need for personal as distinct from professional development to help them to cope.

Box 4.4 Personal problems experienced by medical directors in relation to their posts

- Individual problems
- Reducing the difficulties for medical managers
- Lack of autonomy
- Dealing with difficult medical colleagues
- Gaining acceptability and trust of colleagues
- Managing the dual role of clinician and manager
- Time management
- Financial ability
- Lack of feedback on job performance
- Inadequate financial reward
- Impact on family
- Impact on career

(Reproduced from: Mui Lik D. MPhil Thesis, University of Oxford, 1997.)

Are the core competencies the right ones? Almost certainly not, they are too managerial and do not focus sufficiently on tasks such as stimulating and facilitating clinical change. Current perceptions of development needs are probably wrong because they fix on skills and competencies needed to fulfil current job descriptions. Unfortunately, few organisations have asked if these job descriptions describe the jobs that clinicians really ought to be doing in management. The haphazard way in which clinical director and medical director posts were developed tended to lay too much stress on line management chores while neglecting the real value of medical managers to the process, which is a bridge between medicine and the world of management. If that bridging role is the most important part of the medical manager's job, we need to define the real core competencies to fulfil it. Chief among them is surely clinical credibility, and then the skills of leadership, persuasion, and manipulation; skills associated with acting as a first among equals, as an inspired messenger, and a wise arbiter. These are subtle skills perhaps not teachable, but they are certainly different from budget balancing, purchasing, and personnel management skills, which occupy too much of clinical management time and training.

Personal development

Of course everyone needs to move on in life to evolve and mature. There is nothing new about that. Formalising the activity as "personal development" has, however, become a management fad and I must confess to an heretical aversion to this for it has been an excuse for an almost wholly parasitic service industry to develop to support a fad. Personal development does not mean going to personal development courses; in general personal development, or the honing of generic skills, is a sophisticated process involving targeted education, re-energising through changing job patterns, visiting and sharing with colleagues and, lastly, "mentoring" within or outside one's own organisation. The personal developments needed are inherent in the list of generic skills which clinicians need but which are not formally taught:[33]

- managing yourself (time management)
- managing resources (usually money)
- managing other people: being part of and leading a team;
- managing meetings; appointing and interviewing; giving and taking feedback
- managing knowledge: lifelong learning (including the habit of self-directed learning); writing and publishing; knowledge acquisition skills (libraries and computers); teaching skills.

In the NHS we are not good at facilitating all these forms of personal development. Consultants, in particular, take on jobs like a country parson receiving a living and are expected to carry on a fixed pattern of work with the same momentum throughout life, ministering to the flock on the power of the spiritual lift-off that got them to the job in the first place. It is not enough but it does not mean we need a horde of quasi-professional advisers wanting us to pay them to be wiser than us about what is needed. That is triple jeopardy for the hospital. Pay the manager; pay the guru; pay for a locum. Here is a selection of seminars featured at a personal development show at Olympia in London.

- Downshifting and Career Change.
- Personal Development—Your Competitive Edge.
- Revisioning Your Career.
- Explaining Neuro-Linguistic Programming.
- Dress for Success.
- Downshifting for Positive Life Balance.
- Why Do I Behave The Way I Do.
- Building Your Own Skills Passport.

I confess I did not take a day off work and pay £10 at the door to benefit from all this, it might have been a wonderful life-enhancing experience, but I doubt it. It will certainly have whipped up a lot of business for the business consultants, training providers, counsellors, and "holistic" course providers who sponsored the meeting. Much of the personal development bonanza is a spin-off from the need for people to train "Me plc" to survive in a world of short-term contracts and job mobility; where, as a Department for Education and Employment report found, one-third of employees have never been offered any job training.

The NHS is different. We should manage personal development ourselves within the service and that should be available for all, not just managers. Interviews and questionnaires show that what attracts many people to jobs is the opportunity for further education. A *professional* (as distinct from personal) development within the job ought to be provided routinely by the trust. Beyond that, the sort of mutual support networks and mentoring arrangements that primitive cultures enjoy as routine should be explicitly set up or at least supported. This is particularly important for medical managers, who may feel isolated from their natural peer group and not fully accepted or even supported by other managers. Targeted training for specific skills may be needed and there are outside consultancies who will organise these within NHS institutions. Professional organisations, the King's Fund and the Royal Colleges also arrange short and appropriate training courses. In the future the new NHS University may provide more focused opportunities than are currently accessible. To keep an eye on the evolution of the NHSU log on to http://www.nhsu.nhs.uk.

References

1 Tomlinson Sir B (Chair). *Report of the Inquiry into London's Health Service, Medical Education and Research*. London: HMSO, 1992.
2 Weightman J. Working in teams. In: *Managing People in the Health Service*. London: Institute of Personnel and Development, 1996, pp 36–50.
3 Belbin R. *Management Teams*. Oxford: Butterworth, 1981.
4 Audit Commission. *Medical staffing: a review of national findings*. London. Audit Commission, 2002.
5 National Association of Health Authorities and Trusts (NAHAT). *Hospital and Community Health Services Medical Recruitment Survey*.
6 Finlayson B, Dixon J, Meadows S, Blair G. Mind the Gap: the extent of the NHS Nursing Shortage. *BMJ* 2002;**325**:538–41.
7 Clay B. Flexible training. *BMJ Classified* 23 May:2–3.
8 Audit Commission. *The Doctor's Tale*. London: HMSO, 1995.
9 Young AE. Why Consultants take early retirement and what would stop them. *Bull R Coll Surg Eng* 2002;**84**:230–2.
10 White A, Gatrell J. Appointing SpRs and getting it right first time. *Clin Management* 1997;**6**:9–14.
11 Donaldson L. Conflict, power and negotiation. In: Simpson J, Smith R, eds. *Management for Doctors*. London: BMJ Books, 1995.
12 Honey P. *Problem people*. London: IPD, 1992.
13 Bolton R. *People Skills*. New York: Simon Schuster, 1972.
14 Courtis J. *Bluff Your Way in Management*. Horsham: Ravette Publishing, 1992.
15 Weightman J. *Managing People in the Health Service*. London: Institute of Personnel and Development, 1996.
16 Gatrell J, White T. *Medical Appraisal, Selection and Revalidation*. London: Royal Society of Medicine Press, 2000.
17 Eisenberger R, Cameron J. Detrimental effects of rewards. Reality or myth. *Am Psychol* 1996;**51**:1153–66.
18 Armstrong M. *Managing Rewards Systems*. Milton Keynes: Open University Press, 1993.
19 Bloor K, Maynard A. Rewarding health care teams. *BMJ* 1998;**316**:569.
20 Berne E. *Games People Play*. London: Andre Deutsch, 1966.
21 Macgregor D. *The Human Side of Enterprise*. New York: McGraw-Hill, 1960. (Cited by Weightman J. *Managing People in the Health Service*. London: Institute of Personnel and Development, 1996, p. 120.)
22 McKevitt C, Morgan M. Illness doesn't belong to us. *J Roy Soc Med* 1997;**90**:491–5.
23 Ramirez AJ *et al*. Mental health of hospital consultants, the effects of stress and satisfaction at work. *Lancet* 1996;**347**:724–8.
24 Lindeman S *et al*. A systematic review on gender-specific suicide mortality in medical doctors. *Br J Psychol* 1996;**168**:274–9.
25 Brandon S. *Sick Doctors: a conspiracy of friendliness*. Keele: Mercia, 1995.
26 Seccombe L, Patch A. *Health at Work in the NHS: key indicators. Final Report*. Brighton: Institute of Employment Studies, University of Sussex, 1994.
27 Waldron HA. Sickness in the medical profession. *Ann Occup Hyg* 1996;**40**:391–6.
28 Richards T. Disillusioned doctors. *BMJ* 1997;**314**:1705–6.
29 Caulford PG *et al*. Physician incompetence: specific problems and predictors. *Acad Med* 1993;**270**(Suppl):16–18. (Cited by Holm HA. Quality issues in CME. *BMJ* 1998;**316**:621–4.)

30 Hornick P *et al*. Should business management training be part of medical education? *Ann R Coll Surg Engl* 1997;**79**(Suppl):200–1.
31 Gatrell J, White T. *Medical Student to Medical Director—a development strategy*. NHS Training Division, 1995.
32 Mui Lik D. MPhil Thesis, University of Oxford, 1997.
33 Pencheon D. Development of generic skills. *BMJ* 1998;**316**(Suppl 12):2–3.

5: How the NHS works

> Thus God knows the world because he conceived it in his mind, as if from the outside, before it was created and we do not know its rules, because we live inside it, having found it already made.
>
> (Umberto Eco[1])

I make no apology for including this chapter because if you have now decided to be ordained as a clinical director it's important to have some sense of the theology that underpins the NHS edifice and the intellectual and practical contortions that underpin the dogma as well as understanding the rituals at which you will be expected to officiate.

5.1 Politics, planning, and doctors

The NHS as we are often reminded is one of the world's largest businesses; "as big as the Red Army" they used to say. For those of us inside it is a challenging task trying to see how it works, for it works not just as a structured hierarchical command system like the Red Army but as a subtle, self-motivating, self-adjusting mechanism. Delivering health care to the nation was always so both before and after Aneurin Bevan rebadged it as the National Health Service. The wonder of the NHS is the way in which this adaptation and adjustment occurs. Politicians who have tried to change the NHS radically against the flow of this organic readjustment have found the organism not very biddable. The determinism that rules the NHS is truly organic; by that I mean that there are extensive homeostatic mechanisms quietly at work, repair processes that work effectively without central instruction, even as the parts age, decay or are damaged the whole survives. Indeed, if the totality of central management nationally and locally were to disappear tomorrow the system would remain in responsive, level flight for months or even year; some say it would soar!

The grand axis

By the grand axis of the NHS I mean the defined bureaucratic common structure that transfixes the system from top to bottom which, like the grand axis that transfixed the designs of monumentalist French planners, is intended to give a rationalist's coherence to the whole.

The neat hierarchical "organogram" of the NHS starts at the top with the Secretary for Health as agent of cabinet government and then cascades relentlessly down through the ministers, the NHS Executive, regional outposts, the boards of trusts and through their executive committees to clinical directors and thus to the hapless workers in the service pinned to their desks you might think by the weight of this superstructure. But, of course, it does not work like that—the workers are not hapless, the patients are not passive. True there is a main core of command and control but it is modulated by other forces. That modulation of negative and positive feedback that affects the seemingly simple structure is what creates the stability of the system. More of that later. For the moment we need to consider the basic policymaking forces at work on the central core and the position of doctors in the system.

Formulation of health policy

The formulation of health policy and its execution within the NHS makes a wondrous playground for social scientists and political theorists and for those constructing dead-end courses in minor universities. The complexity and subtlety of the subject confounds accurate or constructive analysis so the field is wide open for historians and theorists; but does all this matter to working doctors and new medical managers? Not really, except that they need to understand that the health policy whose endpoints will embroil them in a lot of sweat, toil, and tears is not the product of a tidy intellectual process where sound facts are processed through a system built to satisfy a clear set of ideological and practical principles. In reality the facts are fragile, as any clinician who has matched the official data to the real will know, and the ideological principles are broad brush: "to supply a comprehensive Health Service open to all free at the point of delivery". Then there is the political reality that the ministers wish to retain their posts and the party wishes to remain in power. Beyond these simple principles and a few political fashions health policies and priorities are a set of compromises between the Department of Health, the Treasury, party ideologues, the BMA, the universities, the Royal Colleges, the patients even. A "complex web of mutual dependencies supporting a shifting assembly of pacts and bargains, both formally negotiated and tacitly understood",[2] or to quote another writer, "policy paradigms are a curious mix of psychological assumptions, scientific concepts, value commitments, social aspirations, personal beliefs and administrative constraints".[3] However capricious policy may eventually seem to the end user, it must, in addition, be formulated within inescapable and constantly fluctuating constraints such as demographic change increasing the numbers of the elderly, European law changing workers' hours, unpredictable economic growth, the arrival of AIDS and immigrants, new technology, fashions in consumer demand, and so on, some quite unexpected and inexplicable, like the seemingly inexorable rise in acute hospital admissions. When one tries to make sense of the policymaking that takes account of all these processes working together, a few threads can be identified which are reasonably consistent, forming what Harrison described as "the shared version of health policy analysis". The major anatomical features of that shared version as summarised and carefully referenced by Harrison et al[4] are as follows.

- Healthcare changes tend to be incrementalist, that is, slow or of narrow scope rather than systematic or radical.
- The policy process is usually one of "partisan mutual adjustment" (PMA) in which no one participant can impose change alone and several can veto it.
- Within the PMA process the medical profession wields enormous influence, however much the politicians of the day may resent that and try to circumvent it.
- The position of lay health authorities and trust board members is weak.
- The position of consumer organisations is even weaker.
- The "Centre" (that is, the Department of Health) has little direct control over the implementation of most national policies.

- The role of managers is usually reactive with the emphasis on "fire fighting", diplomacy, conflict avoidance, and consensus seeking.
- Policy inertia is exacerbated by the complexity of the NHS as a whole.
- The whole complex and slow-moving edifice has been underpinned by an extremely durable political consensus, internally between the government and medical profession, and externally between the government and the people about the primacy of a NHS as an institution.

Whether this cassoulet of diverse ingredients makes for a satisfying and warming dish or an unsatisfactory mush suitable for no one's palate is a matter of taste and expectation, but its various ingredients are crucial to the homeostatic controls that work on the NHS.

Neither Mrs Thatcher nor in his turn Mr Blair liked the taste, so in the infamous *Working for Patients*[5] Mrs Thatcher added piquancy in the shape of market forces, competition, the purchaser/provider split, and fundholding GPs, and Mr Blair gave us *The NHS Plan*.[6] Mrs Thatcher's interventions were unwelcome not only because of their dogmatism and lack of consensuality but also because they disturbed the equilibrium of the system. In addition, crucially, they failed to address the issue of the proper funding of the service, the very pressure that had stimulated the changes. Many of the changes trumpeted in *Working for Patients* were counterproductive to the economic and practical needs of the service. As one commentator observed at the time. "The NHS ... might be seen as the unfortunate victim of a mugging that ought never to have occurred. Saddled at great cost with a market apparatus that nobody really wanted ... it faces a bleak future."[7] Analyses of the effects of "competition" in the NHS show little or no evidence of improved cost effectiveness. This was so even when the direct costs of the internal market were excluded from the equation. Transaction costs in the NHS were about 5% in the 1980s and rose to 12% with the arrival of the internal market.[8,9]

Nevertheless, *Working for Patients* seeded some radical changes in the soil of the NHS culture:

- the concept and the reality that change is possible in the NHS
- change may be implemented quite quickly

- it is feasible and probably preferable to separate the businesses of defining healthcare needs (note that I do not say "purchasing") from the business of providing the care
- the debate about priorities became easier
- the measurement of cost and quality became everyday concerns at all levels in the service.

Despite that, *Working for Patients* slowly worked its way out of agenda papers and into the history books to become just another tuck in the fabric of the service to be replaced by *The NHS Plan*. Certainly, in terms of formulating health policy this had all the hallmarks of consensuality; it followed a short but intense debate about what was needed and the published plan features prominently at its beginning the signatures of 25 top table NHS people, including the presidents of the Royal Colleges of Physicians, of Surgeons, and of GPs, the chair of the British Medical Association, the general secretary of the Royal College of Nursing, and the chief executive of the NHS Confederation. More of *The NHS Plan* later.

The features of NHS policymaking that make for stability also make it difficult to influence, for there is no prince to flatter, no dictator to buy, no chieftain's powwow to attend, no obvious way to change things, so there seems to be an inevitability about most NHS policies when they reach working clinical managers, which tends to imply inalterability. However, this should not deter clinical managers from speaking out—because coherent comment and complaint really does alter the detail when implementing health policy and may contribute to a political environment which eventually allows change. Figure 5.1 shows some examples of the forces at work on the grand axis of central command and which can modulate health policy. Although I have described above the influences as being essentially constructive, there are times when the sheer number of influences working within an organisation as complex as the NHS may frustrate the achievement of *any* endpoint at all, let alone the right one. An example of this is shown in Figure 5.2, which is the chart Dr Susan Atkinson constructed to try to understand the forces at work in medical manpower planning following the establishment of LMWAGs (Local Medical Workforce Advisory Groups) in 1996. The details are not all now correct but the Byzantine patchwork remains true of this and many other systems in the NHS.

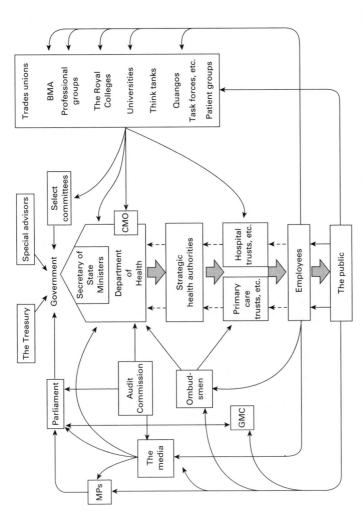

Figure 5.1 Simplified diagram of the pressures acting on decision-making processes in the NHS.

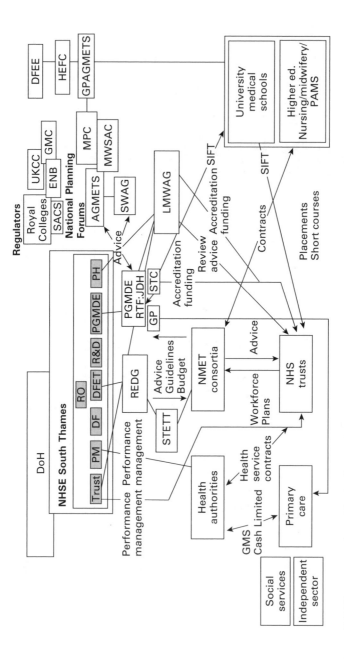

Figure 5.2 Diagram produced by Dr Susan Atkinson to help the newly formed LMWAG (Local Medical Workforce Advisory Group) understand the LMWAG "in the context of regional and national bodies and processes focused on aspects of service planning and workforce supply". There is no need to define the acronyms used here. The figure is intended merely to bemuse.

In the midst of all this it is worth looking more closely at the relationship between the government/Department of Health and the medical profession, because it is that relationship which threw up the principle that clinicians in management are "a good thing"; and it is problems with that relationship which causes so much of the angst that erodes morale within the service.

Relationships between government and doctors

As I conceive it the function of the Ministry of Health is to provide the medical profession with the best and most modern apparatus of medicine, and to enable them freely to use it, in accordance with their training, for the benefit of the people of this country. Every doctor must be free to use that apparatus without interference from secular organisations.

(Ernest Bevin in the House of Commons 30/4/46 *Hansard* Col. 52)

Starting with the deals that Aneurin Bevan made with the doctors at the inception of the NHS in 1946, there was for 50 years an unspoken pact between the profession and a sequence of governments and the Department of Health. The culture of the pact was that the government/Department of Health would act centrally to set the political agenda and define the funding available, but would leave the peripheral side of the business to the doctors who would decide how best to deliver care, how to respond to changes in medical advances, and even deal with politically sensitive issues such as rationing. In the last 10 years that pact has taken a beating and it is worth questioning whether it still exists.

The more political or less kind social scientists have interpreted the profession's stance in this compact with the government as being essentially self protective, defensive, conservative, and cynical—frustrating all moves that might diminish the profession's power, influence or income and one could argue that in spite of all their protestations to the contrary this is the belief which underpins many of the Blair government reforms. Doctors themselves, in contrast, see their public role as being the sole protectors of patients against a succession of governments bent only on controlling cost and imposing dogma. The doctor as "mother tiger". Both these views can, of course, be true! What is certain is that there has always been a degree of what social scientists call "liberal corporatism".[10] Liberal corporatism describes a process in which to ease the business of running complex organisations the government abrogates responsibilities for some of its tasks to certain moderate and well-organised groupings who it can expect to control their members and liaise constructively with the public. The medical profession is one such and of course even now remains so. Government regulatory agencies such as CHAI and the NCAA are predominantly staffed by doctors.

Until the late 1970s the marriage was acceptably harmonious, free of too many arguments about money, even though as early as 1953 a committee had been set up to try to control expenditure on the NHS. Money has since then been the root of all difficulties. Firstly, dramatically, in the late 1970s when doctors questioned the government's stewardship of the budget not only in relation to their own salaries but also in terms of the allocation for health care itself. This was eventually brought to the brink of "industrial action". Although the salaries issue was, to some extent, resolved the general funding of the NHS has never really been determined. The principles of cash limits and resource allocation did not resolve the problem nor did the importation of managerialism as a consequence of the Griffiths Report of 1983.[11] To control costs the government had to make inroads into areas which the traditional compact had left to doctors. Managers cannot alone control costs and where costs continually outrun the supply of money, doctors (who are usually the first and the loudest in complaint) are perceived as the agents of overspending. In taking over areas previously left to doctors the attack was on two fronts, both of which were based on the principle that it is doctors who commit resources and spend money.

1. The basis on which they do this must be questioned—hence evidence-based medicine and managed care (*see* Section 6.8, "Audit, evidence-based medicine, and managed care").
2. Doctors must be "on board" so that they understand the finite nature of available funds and take direct managerial responsibility for the use of those funds—hence the clinical director.

Therefore with the arrival of clinical directors and fundholding GPs there was born a new and formal extension of the longstanding pact of liberal corporatism. The principle was that an elite of doctors could be recruited to deliver budget targets and bring pressure to bear in controlling costs in areas such as length of stay, use of drugs, application of new technology, etc.

The NHS Plan

With clinical management structures firmly in place it was clear by the beginning of the Blair government's time in office that these exercises had not solved the resource problems of the NHS, had not mollified public dissatisfaction, and furthermore the scandals of Bristol paediatric heart surgery, Alder Hay, and Harold Shipman gave ammunition to the view that health care could not be entrusted to doctors. Three things were perceived as necessary: more money, a change in culture, and as a corollary to raise the chances of success, more control.

If you read *The NHS Plan* (it is in fact quite readable!) it states unequivocally that:

> In part the NHS is failing to deliver because over the years it has been underfunded. In particular there have been too few doctors and nurses and other key staff to carry out all the treatments required. But there have been other underlying problems as well. The NHS is a 1940s system operating in a 21st century world. It has:
>
> a lack of national standards
> old fashioned demarcations between staff and barriers between services
> a lack of clear incentives and levers to improve performance
> over centralization and disempowered patients.

The NHS Plan was bold in its scope: 7000 extra beds, 100 new hospitals, 7500 more consultants and 2000 more GPs, 20 000 extra nurses, and the Chancellor duly raised taxes to pay the expected cost. The reform to current practice that was asked for as the *quid pro quo* involves the establishment of performance frameworks and regulatory agencies to police them, a Modernisation Board and a £500 million performance fund to encourage and spread good practice and so on. *The NHS Plan* also says:

> Local hospitals cannot be run from Whitehall. There will be a new relationship between the Department of Health and the NHS to enshrine the trust that patients have for frontline staff. The principle

of subsidiarity will apply. A new system of earned autonomy will devolve power from the centre to the local health service as modernisation takes hold.

The broad intent of *The NHS Plan* was to "modernise" the NHS and transform it from its technocratic, paternalistic design into a consumer responsive "patient-centred" service. This was an extension of the Blairite "third way" policy to the NHS and was said to combine central direction with local autonomy, sanctions with reward, central planning with competition at the local level. Ham described "The Third Way" in health care as being "eclectic and pragmatic" but essentially just a rhetorical device which failed to recognise the complexity of steering mechanisms required in a public service.[12] The potentially schizophrenic effect of wanting more central control yet allowing more front-line freedom has been recognised, but the two are not incompatible: freedom is merely seen as something desirable but nevertheless not something allowing license for poor performance. To ensure this there must be supervision. Even the Secretary of State is said to be aware of the dangers in this and Cabinet Office papers are reported as recognising that "excessively directive methods of government that appear to treat front-line deliverers as unable to think for themselves, untrustworthy or incompetent, undermine the very motivation and adaptability on which real-world success depends".[13]

One of the unspoken corollaries of *The NHS Plan* is that it implies that the NHS may be managed out of its problems. Although *The NHS Plan* waxes lyrical about the number of extra doctors and nurses it will employ, it is silent on the huge number of extra managers that are being recruited to achieve its ends and equally silent on the huge risk that such overmanagement entails. Since 1995 the number of senior managers in the NHS has increased by 24% and by September 2001 there were 269 080 managers and support staff, compared to 266 170 nurses.

The obsession with control

The combined effect of the near total dependence of health service funding on central taxes distributed through the Treasury, which ensures a continuing and desperate search for financial stability, with the belief that frontline professionals are the agents of wilful and inappropriate spending coupled with a loss of respect for the autonomy of professional groups, has trapped recent governments into an ever-tightening demand for control while publicly sounding off about devolvement of power. This is politely described as the move from "public administration" to "public management". As with traditional administration, public management is often offered as a set of neutral reforms for increasing the efficiency and responsiveness of public service delivery in a more complex economic and social environment. However, as several writers have argued, this perspective should be regarded with suspicion, not least because public management carries with it its own set of values and assumptions which if cultural change is to be achieved may be used to supplant those of the administrative cultures it seeks to replace or control.[14] Simon Jenkins in his book, *Accountable to None*,[15] documented in detail the development of this trend during the years of Thatcherite government driven by a relentless desire for cost savings. In that quest any financial risk was to be minimised and the delegation to the periphery and to professionals by which the service had previously been managed became suspect. As Jenkins remarks:

> The act of delegation requires the delegator to take risks, especially in the short term. Yet politics is about minimizing risk, avoiding bad publicity, watching out for banana skins. By centralizing decision, a minister can give himself the illusion that he is minimizing risk. He may be but he is blanketing decision in a fog of caution and irresolution.

The desire to control—the old Stalinist reflex of governments of all colours—is not reflected in good management practice in the world outside which stresses the importance of empowering the functional units within an organisation, giving them leeway in achieving or even exceeding the corporate objectives. The consequence of a demand for control is a crippling bureaucracy, the issuing of directives without proper consultation and the endless demand for "returns", reams of neurotically collected data attempting to ensure that directives are being observed: even at one point "how many managers do you have?", "how much do they cost?", "how are you going to reduce their numbers?" This last was indeed the ultimate irony in that the mouth wanted to bite the hand it commissioned to feed it! Meanwhile, as Jenkins ruefully concluded in his chapter on the NHS in the time of the Thatcher government:

> the centralization of the service left an uneasy feeling that a professional relationship of trust between patient and doctor and hospital and community had been broken. A new and cruder accountability had been put in place, to a vague concept of national efficiency and to a nervous minister to parliament.

Perceiving the failure first of a bureaucratised management and then of clinical management to transform the health service, the Blair government's *The NHS Plan*, as we have seen, further tightened the screw of control by constructing a national performance management edifice. This consists of setting national standards, promulgating national service frameworks, and then policing them. To do this the government added five national regulatory agencies into the already overcrowded field: NICE, CHAI, NCAA, the National Patient Safety Agency, and the Modernisation Agency. The evolution of this extension of central regulation will be interesting to watch. Walshe has pointed out that regulation can go down two routes, deterrence or compliance, and that studies of regulation show that a responsive approach matching style of regulation to the organisation under scrutiny is the better policy.[16] To achieve this regulators need three virtues:

- *knowledge*, which is the prerequisite for respect
- *power*, so they are taken seriously
- *independence*, so that they can be trusted by those they seek to regulate.

In the context of the NHS, independence is unlikely to be granted yet curiously ministers go out of their way to claim that their new plans encaspsulate a "shift of power to the front line" and they claim this forcefully and, one would like to think, with honesty. The thesis seems to be that with firm regulation you can let go of the other controls. However, seasoned observers note that this freedom is illusory and most likely to be in the form of rather vague rewards for those who comply with central direction. At the time of writing, the highest of these rewards will be "Foundation Status" entitling hospitals to set their own pay rates and borrow money for capital projects. The same sort of benefits were promised when trust hospitals were first established but no real freedoms were ever apparent. The foundation hospitals may well end up with what Klein calls a "cacophony of accountabilities"[17] as they struggle to reconcile their own internal needs and aspirations with those of a Department of Health that has not really given up control and a third force, which emerges whenever "social ownership" is put in place as it will be with foundation hospitals. That third force will be the board of governors, which will be a mix of "the public", patients, employees, and "partner organisations" such as primary care trusts. Oh yes, and there will also be a fourth finger in the pie, that of the "independent regulator".

Historians amongst you may note that a lot of this is scarily reminiscent of the structure of the old Soviet economy with the "constant repetition of shibboleths ('core values'), the flow of diktats, the abrupt and unexpected changes in direction and even the show trials in which doctors and managers are publicly humiliated".[18] If you are too young to remember all that you can comfort yourself by viewing all this control as simply a shift in society's attitude to the means by which public services are accountable. You might also hope that the concept of standard setting and central performance management is sound and will deliver better quality services. Whatever your view, the fact is that any compact such as it was between government and professions hardly exists any more and clinical directors are at risk of becoming merely "pigs in the middle" between the controller and the controlled.

The clinical director as "piggy in the middle"

Historians may, in due course, record the failure of clinical management. If they do so it may be because we have tried to load clinical managers with three further objectives in addition to the control of expenditure. The other targets being delivery of quantity, quality, and compliance. Unfortunately, these requirements are frequently irreconcilable, and by attempting to reconcile the delivery of quality, quantity, and compliance with centrally set standards at a specific cost volunteer clinical directors may come close to extinction as a breed and the compact between the government and the profession will need to be reworked yet again.

There are, no doubt, those who say that the power of doctors should and can be curtailed so that no further compact is necessary. The power of doctors has in essence always been the possession of the magic of medicine. Only they can say the spells and only they occupy what has been called "the secret garden". The automation of clinical management by EBM-driven protocols and the steady denigration of professionalism by those outside has not yet, as Klein claimed, shrunk the secret garden to the size of a window box.[19] Despite the rise in complaints and litigation, surveys show that patients still believe that doctors are more likely to look after their interests than are managers or politicians; so long as that perception remains, the magicians will need to be given a place.

The current or a future government may wish to let the imposition of financial imperatives and centrally defined standards of care force the pace and may not bother to make accommodations with the profession; but this seems unlikely. At the very least it will need to take into account the views of medical managers, particularly if those managers can show themselves to be cognisant and sympathetic to the realities of running an effective health service. If medical managers remains an entity in the NHS they are likely to define and lead the professional end of any continued compact.

One should not leave this arena on too sour a note. The management of the NHS has been bedevilled by its very complexity, its size, the lack of adequate data about how it is working and what it needs to do, confounded by unremitting and ungovernable change. It is reasonable to suppose that even had it been undertaken by different people to different rules the results would have been much the same or worse.

5.2 NHS finance

What a tragedy it is to live in an age of such consummate cost consciousness.

(Bill Bryson[20])

As medical managers you will spend too much time explaining to staff that although you deprecate the continuing shortage of money in the NHS and understand their desires for more, there is nothing you yourself can do to increase that sum of money, and they will need to grapple with the reality that whatever the Chancellor of the Exchequer might promise there is nevertheless a finite budget. It is not an argument you will enjoy promulgating but you will do it so often that it is helpful to know enough of NHS finances to understand why things are as they are.

Where the money comes from

The money which funds the NHS comes predominantly from general taxation, with a much lesser contribution from the National Insurance scheme, a fraction from prescription charges, small amounts from private practice within NHS institutions, and miscellaneous sources such as the sale of land. The majority thus comes directly from the Exchequer. The sums involved are huge and represent about 14% of public spending which itself represents 43% of the gross domestic product (GDP = what we earn as a nation + what as a nation we borrow [PSBR (public sector borrowing requirement)]). Forty years ago NHS expenditure as a percentage of GDP was a mere 3%. It reached 7% as the new century arrived and is scheduled to rise further (Figure 5.3). Nevertheless, in times of difficulty all of us within the NHS like to point out that the NHS still claims a smaller percentage of GDP than almost all our Western European colleagues and about half of what is claimed in the USA. A public health guru or sage Treasury official might respond that the quality or even the quantity of care that the money buys in the UK is, in fact, comparable to that in equivalent countries, and that many health indices, such as access to basic care, life expectancy, and perinatal mortality, are better in the UK than in comparable countries. But at what cost? An overworked, abused, and deprofessionalised workforce still demoralised by the insufficiency of finance *vis-à-vis* a decent environment for them and their patients; a slow, inadequate response to advances in health care; real and continuing deficiencies in psychiatric and community care and extensive covert rationing—all of this made more irritating by the seeming

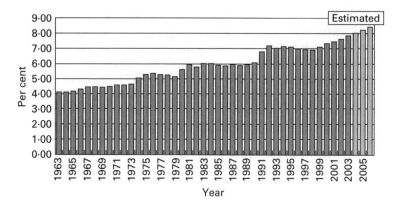

Figure 5.3 UK NHS spending as a percentage of the GDP (gross national product) 1963–2006. (From *Health Care UK 2001*, King's Fund; reproduced with permission.)

non-appearance or disappearance of money promised by the government.

From their insulated fastnesses the public health theoretician and the Treasury official may continue to conclude that funding is adequate, but the perception from the front line is that it is not. Although national surveys show the majority of UK citizens are generally very content with "their" health service the percentage who are dissatisfied has stayed depressingly constant and probably more swayed by the fluctuating stance of the media than by actual experience (Figure 5.4). International comparators, however, show that there is a relationship between the spending per head on health care and the users' satisfaction (Figure 5.5).

How the money is allocated

There are two sides to NHS finance: the allocation of money, "the *supply* side"; and the demands for its use, "the *demand* side."

In defining the supply side the government is subject to the general political pressures on it. Education and health are usually in fashion, defence is not. Social security is not in fashion, quite the opposite, but it is largely uncontrollable and is the greatest demand on the public purse. The annual exercise in settling the total amount available to the NHS, in

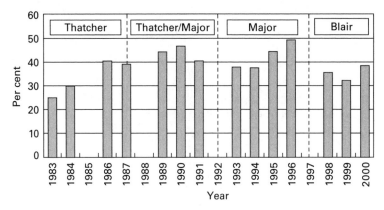

Figure 5.4 Dissatisfaction with the NHS: percentage stating very or quite dissatisfied, 1993–2000. (From *Health Care UK 2001*, King's Fund; reproduced with permission.)

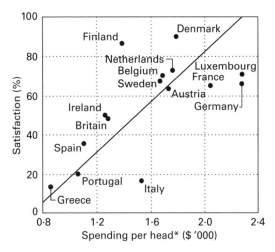

Figure 5.5 Health spending and public satisfaction with health services. *AV purchasing power parity

theory, takes account of medical advances, the funding implications of government policies as well as inflation, but the allocations for these are rarely what the real figures would demand (Figure 5.6), and there is a further reducing effect in that a percentage is also removed for anticipated "productivity

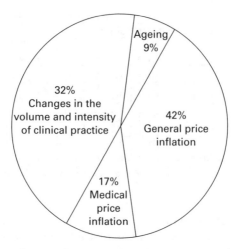

Figure 5.6 Contribution of separate factors to the increase in healthcare spending. (Data source: Muir Gray, *Evidence-Based Healthcare*; Figure 2.5.)

gains". This productivity gain is expected to be made every year, which leaves the Treasury with a happy prospect that some time during this century the cost of providing health care will approach zero!

Once the overall sum for the year is allocated to the NHS it is deemed to be fixed. In the jargon the service is "cash limited". However, within the service itself not all budgets are cash limited. Hospital services are, but GP prescribing is currently not. Once the total is agreed centrally the central costs of running the NHS are deducted and the remainder distributed to health authorities, although some is "top sliced" for special areas such as HIV, cancer, and other pet projects. The mechanics of allocation to regions, and within regions to specific districts and trusts, is determined by complex formulae, the validity and application of which are hotly argued by those who see themselves as doing badly as a result of the allocations; which is pretty much everybody. The mechanics of allocation change regularly in an attempt to make it simpler or more equitable. Since 1990 the process has been one of resident/capitation-based funding. Each region's population is "weighted" to reflect the age profile within the region and the demands that its population place on the NHS. These "capitation rates" are based on the estimated expenditure per head for different age groups. The age-weighted populations are adjusted by the SMR (standardised mortality ratio) and social deprivation and certain geographical supplements are then added, such as "London weighting" to reflect the higher costs for staff living in the capital. The derivation of the formulation and its application is modified to some extent by political considerations and the difficulty of taking money from one part of the country to give to another. Academics who deal in these matters are never satisfied and Sheldon has pointed out that, in fact, the use of a much simpler formula based simply on population size, age and SMR would be just as good.[21] The rules governing allocation are reasonably fixed but latitude in them allows for separate districts to feel hard done by. Poor and deprived areas seem always to lose out. The position of teaching trusts is also disputed. Those outside, of course, consider them over resourced so a detailed dissection of teaching hospital costs is done to separate the costs of teaching and of research from those of service to make them more explicit and thus more accountable. Unfortunately, as anyone in a teaching hospital knows, the three faces of teaching hospital medicine are so intricately interwoven that no accurate division is achievable, and dissection shows the whole body to be starved rather than obese.

Allocations are rendered even more opaque by the top slicing of money for specific areas such as educational budgets from which trainees are partly paid. After all this the money is then, of course, not allocated directly to the provider units but to the purchasers who go round another complex set of exercises as part of the contracting process which decides who will do what and who gets the money. In this, the third turn of the merry-go-round, cost and quality of service are taken into account and purchasing is also used as a vehicle to force changes in the configuration of providers, to encourage mergers, etc. The process is summarised in Figure 5.7.

The complex rules controlling this fairground may mean that money targeted for particular front-line projects may never reach them. For example, in 2002 Professor Mike Richards, the "Cancer Tsar" had to admit that of £255 million earmarked for the cancer plan in 2001 almost none had reached the front line. Yes, that is right, a quarter of a billion pounds had disappeared, and worse than that, Department of

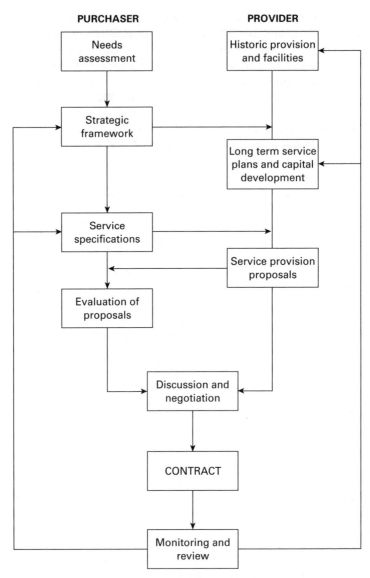

Figure 5.7 Cross-relationships between purchasers and providers in the contracting process.

Health officials had no idea where it had gone! Targeted funding, it seems, comes in three sorts: "hypothecated", "earmarked", and "ring fenced" (in increasing order of firmness as to where it is intended to go). The cancer money probably disappeared to pay the debts of the health authorities or trusts that were way stations between the Department of Health and the cancer teams. What is really depressing is that they were entirely within their rights as only earmarked funds must go where they are intended!

The trail from tax-payers' pockets via the Treasury, Department of Health, NHS Executive, and purchasers to the hospitals that care for them is more convoluted than the ways drug barons use to launder their proceeds. There is thus no way that any medical managers would be able to justify to their staff whether or not the budget they are working to represents a fair allocation. There must be simpler ways, but the simplest and most transparent, such as the "fee for item of service" which is much put about by disenchanted staff, is unacceptable because that mechanism takes away the ability to manipulate and to cash limit the service.

One should not deny the importance of getting allocation right, both at a macro and a micro level. Thomas Getzen, a US health economist, says that in health economics "Allocation, Allocation, Allocation" is what is important, echoing the estate agent's priority "Location, Location, Location".[22] If the *right patient*, is going to get the *right treatment* in the *right place* at the *right time*, allocation needs to be accurate, adequate, and forceful. The NHS tends to fall down on all three.

Why can't more money be raised?

So long as the government of the day believes that the efficiency and productivity of the NHS is substandard and could be improved, and it believes it can weather the little squalls about health that constantly blow through the media, there is no incentive radically to review the funding basis of the NHS. Each new government is encouraged to review the mechanics of funding but never does. If it were to, what options would it have?

- A rise in general taxation levels.
- An hypothecated tax, that is, one earmarked for health.
- A reallocation of spending from other ministries to health.
- Increased and new charges for services, for example £10 for visiting a GP, £25 a day for time in hospital.
- Withdrawal of funding from health care, retreating to a safety net for the poor or to an emergencies-only service.
- Part payment, leaving enforced personal insurance to pick up the remainder of the cost.

None of these, of course, commends itself and the option of money from the National Lottery, makes but a tiny dimple in the problem. Interestingly, the public is not as averse to changes in the funding of the NHS as you would think, it is insiders who are more likely to revere the founding principle of a free service. A Mori poll in 1998 commissioned by Age Concern showed that three-quarters of those polled still believed in a free NHS, but 39% thought that those who failed to follow medical advice should not receive free treatment and 44% thought non-essential items should be covered by insurance rather than the NHS. No government has yet shown any sign of withdrawal from the full commitment to the NHS. Each government therefore falls back on the only real option remaining to it, namely a bit more money but primarily cost containment in the historical certainty that almost any extra funding is quickly swallowed in line with Parkinson's Second Law that "expenditure rises to meet income" and that complaints of underfunding are only temporarily assuaged because demand seems to be inexorable (Figure 5.8).

Demand

The government sees the outputs of the healthcare process continually rising, more people are treated year on year, but these outputs fall short of *demand* which is almost certainly short of, or at least different from, *need*. The need for health care, far from diminishing as Bevan hoped in 1947, has grown. NHS activity has risen from seven million FCEs (finished consultant episodes) in 1990 to 12·2 million in 1999/2000. All this of course probably represents not a sicker population but simply changed expectations of health.

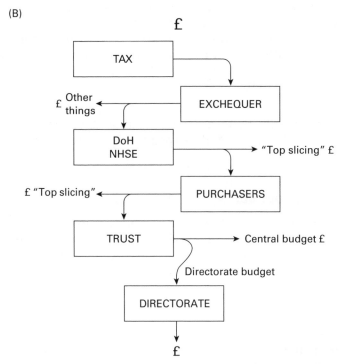

Figure 5.8 (A) Options for breaking into the taxation–allocation–provision cycle. (B) Laundering the tax-payers' money. No one working in a clinical directorate can judge the fairness of allocation because of the complexity of the process.

Accident and Emergency attenders rose from 36 million in 1990 to 43 million in 2000 and the number of outpatient attenders increased from 10·8 million in 1995/96 to 13·5 million in 1999/2000. The General Household Survey of 1996/97, when compared to that of 1972, showed a doubling in the percentage of the population who categorise themselves as suffering from an acute illness.

Behind all this lurks the waiting list, so beloved by the media as an indicator and still standing at well over one million. It will always be impossible to match financial inputs to health outputs for a variety of reasons. For example:

- new technology usually yields less health gain per £ spent than does old technology (Figure 5.9)
- despite all the effort by government and hospitals, the real productivity of cases treated per £ spent has fallen
- shorter hours for doctors in training, less service work from them, new technology, much more time spent in bureaucratic activities, increased contact time with patients, hours spent in often futile audit are all lowering real productivity.

Quite simply, there are more staff and yet we see less patients each per year and we spend more money on each one of them.

Hidden unmet costs

A worrying feature of the NHS that budget-holding managers will quickly discover is an invisible line in the budget. It should be there and should include the costs thus far unmet of "backlog maintenance" plus the cost of obviating clinical and other risks already known about and the cost of replacing equipment that is obsolete but for which there is no replacement plan. There are other things to add here but these are the big three. No figure exists for the national total in this invisible line. An NHS Confederation Survey released in 1998 concluded that at least £3 billion was needed just for essential maintenance and it's probably much more now. It's one of those bottomless sink holes into which "new money" disappears.

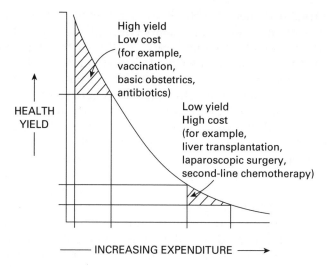

Figure 5.9 Higher levels of expenditure on health services do not normally produce as much health gain per £ as do lower levels.

Revenue, capital, and capital charges

Revenue is the day-to-day housekeeping money that is spent on patient care. *Capital* is the separately allocated sum used for large items of expenditure; strictly defined as anything capable of being used for more than a year and costing more than £5000, so all buildings and most equipment are *capital*. The capital budget is allocated to trusts and districts and some is retained centrally.

The mechanics of allocation and expenditure also have to take into account depreciation and are just as complex as the processes for allocating revenue. Trusts are required to pay back notional interest on capital to ensure efficiency in its use so that, for example, we do not hang on to empty buildings or have more pieces of equipment than are needed. It is, in short, to ensure that we "sweat our assets". It was also once perceived by many as a Conservative government's first steps towards "privatisation" of the NHS. In the NHS capital cannot, in theory, be used as revenue and vice versa.

The issue of the financing of the NHS will remain, as it always has been, an unedifying and untidy spectacle. The government desperate to limit costs will avoid talking about inputs and talk about outputs. Government spokespeople will always talk about how many more of this or that have been dealt with in the last year without observing whether that met need. Providers will only fix on the outputs they might provide if finance were sufficient and purchasers will try to win all the outputs they think they need for the input that has been allocated. Battles will be fought largely in the media. It is, as Klein has observed, a "dialogue of the deaf". In the same essay, Klein goes on to point out that any narrative on the NHS will always "revert to the built in tensions that spring directly from the original failure to base the funding of the NHS on anything more solid than the shifting sands of political fashions and governmental preferences". A failure which would, he predicts, allow him "to describe a climax in which the curtain comes down on the NHS in financial flames". Instead he says there is "no *gotterdammerung*—but a final anticlimax as the firemen led by … the secretary of state rush onto the stage to douse the fire with buckets of money in the last act".[23] He wrote that describing the NHS of the 1980s, but it is no less true of the NHS of the twenty-first century except that the fireman is now the prime minister and the bucket is much bigger.

PFI (private finance initiative)

The continuing, very public, twist to this tale of funding the NHS is the continuing saga of PFI, the private finance initiative. This is an initiative not solely directed at changing the way NHS capital projects are funded but is also being applied throughout the public services. The thesis, simplified, goes like this. We need a new hospital/hospital building, etc. We do not have the capital and we know that even if we did we are inefficient at arranging for buildings to go up to budget and on time. So let us get the more efficient private sector to put up the building, service it, and have a lease on it. We will just pay them annually for the use of that resource or even better will give them our spare land or buildings in exchange and/or let them provide the support services that are needed in the hospital. All the NHS now has to do is rent space for our doctors and nurses to treat patients in. It truly encapsulates the "enjoy now pay later philosophy" of the end of the twentieth century. It is much more complicated than that, of course, but the underlying thesis seemed sound and there was the encouraging prospect of consortia of financiers, builders and service specialists working together to do their own things well for the NHS.

Unfortunately, the process has been fraught with difficulties, many of which are complex but all of which have conspired to prevent the majority of projects going ahead. Five examples will suffice.

Scale

Overall, there were too many schemes. The initiative was intended to "let a thousand flowers bloom" but, of course, capital and backers and those capable of delivering were limited, so the number of projects has been curtailed but is still very substantial and far outside what traditional state funding might have afforded. The scale of the projects' costs has escalated and analysis shows that in many instances the cost of achieving the objective using public money would have been less than if it was left to PFI consortia. Gaffney and Pollock studied 14 such projects and found that during development the estimated cost of the schemes rose by an average of 72%.[24]

Alison Pollock has been a brave, professional, and unrelenting analyst of the PFI process and to update yourself on it you could usefully conduct a literature search on her name or start at the BMJ web reference for her 2002 paper[25] and follow the debate from the from there with the links.

Unrealistic expectations of performance

Efficiency savings are often required in the use of the new buildings if the package is to be affordable, but these savings are often untested or unachievable. The Edinburgh Royal Infirmary Scheme, for example, anticipated a 35% increase in patient throughput per bed.

Risk transfer

Risk transfer was inherent in the original PFI concept. The consortia would, in theory, carry part of the risk of future changes in work patterns, care purchasing, building regulations, etc. The consortia, however, realised that almost all these issues are under government control and that therefore the government should bear more of the risk. This, known as the "ultra vires" issue, remains to be resolved to everyone's satisfaction, even though the NHS Private Finance Act of 1997 addressed it directly.

There is no such thing as free money

All PFI projects are an impending debt on the public purse merely deferring current capital expenditure and replacing it by an increased current expenditure bill in the future; yet the Accounting Standards Board has been unable thus far to persuade the Treasury that these PFI projects need to be included in the PSBR (public sector borrowing requirement) and PFI companies have used cunning accounting practices to keep their own debt off the companies' balance sheets.

Employee considerations

One of the factors inherent in most PFI schemes is the provision of non-clinical labour by the PFI partner. In many instances this may simply involve transferring the lowest paid NHS employees to a different employer, potentially for a lower wage or into different conditions of employment. The unions regard this, of course, with considerable suspicion and the process has been bedevilled by uncertainty about "TUPE" (the transfer of undertakings [protection of employment]). The trades unions are understandably unhappy about the effect of PFI on their members.

These and other problems lead one to consider whether PFI is really as good as once we thought. Can we really afford the uncertain future costs of PFI? There is after all, as the man said, "no such thing as a free lunch". Medical managers caught up in all this need to remain very sanguine and not to get too carried away by the exciting prospect of a seemingly free new hospital! If you are involved in the planning phase of a PFI scheme make sure the specification is comprehensive and covers what you will need. Take a simple example. Your PFI partner is required in the contract to provide car parking and you specify how many places you want. On that specification all you will get is the cheapest option, that is, a concrete slab.

Do you want it lit? Fenced? Barriers? Security provided? Entry control arrangements? Billing for staff users? If so you will only get them if you draw the original contract very tightly. It is a simple example and you might scold me for stating the obvious. But it happens. Haringey Borough Council committed itself to a PFI plan to refurbish its schools, only to discover that it had forgotten to specify that furniture and equipment would be needed in these schools. A lapse that cost £6 million. PFI "partners" are not charities and are unlikely to point out your lapses of concentration to you.

5.3 Top to bottom: NHS management structures and how they work

To the newcomer there is often confusion about who does what and who is accountable to whom in the hierarchy of the NHS. It is a topic where clear definitions are rare and where the actual dynamics only rarely reflect the ideal. To get a feel for how the upper tiers of the system are structured power up your computer, connect to the internet and go to http://www.doh.gov.uk/about and travel on from there. You may find the experience informative or you may find it worryingly Kafkaesque. There is a warning hint of this on the Department of Health home page. "The NHS is not part of the DoH" it says.

Start again! This time go to http://www.nhs.uk/thenhsexplained/how_the_nhs_works.asp where, among other statements, you will find that the Department of Health is responsible for:

- management of the overall health … system
- developing policy and managing major change in the NHS
- regulation and inspection of the NHS
- intervention should problems occur at any stage in the NHS.

Most of us do not have the time for this sort of *quodlibet* so to abbreviate it let us just note that essentially the hierarchy in what you and I would call the NHS looks like this (Figure 5.10).

This is very simplified. There are for instance many other agencies, such as the Medicines Control Agency, that are directly

Figure 5.10 Organogram of the NHS.

controlled by the Department of Health as are CHAI and NICE. There are also some special health authorities which serve the needs of the whole kingdom, such as the National Blood Transfusion Service. Additionally, there are multitudinous other side branches adorned with advisory bodies and think tanks, professional panels, steering groups, liaison committees, focus groups, and advisors, but for all this there is fundamentally a straight line chain of responsibility between individual doctors and the Secretary of State. With each government's reforms there is an expectation and a promise that "front-line staff" will gain significant independence from previous hierarchical controls. In reality no great differences are encountered.

Ministers

The Secretary of State is responsible to Parliament for the functions and functioning of the NHS. To assist him in this he has ministers, currently five. These are of lower profile and have specific areas of concern. Although the Secretary of State and Ministers are advised by the Department of Health, the Chief Medical Officer, and so on, they are politicians and their horizons rarely extend beyond the next election. Also, because their concerns come to us through the distorting lens of the media we tend to hear their views crudely put. As medical managers struggling to get things done, it is easy to be upset by the pronouncements of ministers; we should not be, they are not intended for us. There is often, however, a streak of more than just performance art in the minister's show; there may truly be some self delusion. Amanda Mitchison commented at the end of her interview with Baroness Jay, one time Minister of Health in the Lords:

> we seem to have been talking about two quite different health services. The NHS you and I know is a place of crumbling buildings, and long waits, and understaffing, and bureaucracies busy robbing Peter to just about pay Paul—and yet, for all that, it still remains, on the whole, pretty good. The grot is just part of the British experience ... An undeniable fact of existence. But not in Margaret Jay's book. Her hospitals are brimming with eager beavers and exciting initiatives and optimistic, can-do martinets on greater efficiency drives. This is the world as presented so often to us by politicians, limitless possibilities on no more cash. Never acknowledge, never concede, refute the irrefutable. They must take us for such fools.[26]

In due course Baroness Jay was promoted to full cabinet rank and turned her attentions to "modernising" the House of Lords.

Do not worry. What really matters is that the advice ministers get is as sound as possible and that in your turn you listen only to what is actually planned to happen; that will be finalised not in Westminster but will emerge as papers from the Department of Health or one of its pseudopodia, distilled as another ubiquitous *Executive Letter* or *Health Service Circular*. If you are in management long enough, you will be able to enjoy the hobby of matching circulars that reflect in a deadpan way governments' about turns. Competition one year, cooperation the next, care in the community one year, care in hospital another.

The Department of Health, by the way, is not unaudited. The Public Accounts Committee, the Audit Commission, and of course the Treasury, keep a beady and possibly jaundiced eye on it. There is also the Health Service Commissioner or Ombudsman to watch out for "maladministration".

At the Department of Health, board members include the chief executive, the chief medical and chief nursing officers, the directors of finance, communication, research, human resources, and so on—just like your own trust board. An offshoot of the board currently is the Modernisation Board overseeing the Modernisation Agency that will "act as the 'centre for Excellence' in identifying and celebrating good practice in the NHS and demonstrating how 'know how' can be spread across the whole Service" it will "also develop current and future NHS leaders and managers at all levels in the NHS and all health professionals".

The chief medical officer

The CMO (chief medical officer) is a high profile job and doctors often ask where this post fits into the management hierarchy. The CMO is not strictly in the managerial chain though he or she is on the NHS board. In essence, their task is to be the medical senior advisor to the Secretary of State as well as to other government bodies. The CMO is effectively the Director of Public Health for England. That a previous CMO, Sir Kenneth Calman, had his name attached to two initiatives, the "Calmanisation" of training and the Calman–Hine proposals for cancer services, illustrates the centrality of the role in planning.

Strategic health authorities

The strategic health authorities "are responsible for developing strategies for the local health services and ensuring high quality performance. They manage the NHS and also ensure that national priorities (such as programmes for improving cancer services) are integrated into local plans".

Trust structures

There is, of course, more to the NHS than trusts, but a description of trusts will serve to illustrate typical mechanics. We have already seen that there are usually three tiers of management in trusts: a board, an executive group, both of which are responsible for the whole organisation, and below that subgroupings typically called clinical directorates, that manage the day-to-day business of particular services, surgery, pathology, critical care, whatever.

The board

The trust board mimics to some extent the board of any commercial company, with its chairperson, NEDs (non-executive directors), and executive members. The board of an NHS trust is a statutory body with its membership prefigured. There is a chairperson, appointed by the Secretary of State. Chairs are usually lay people but with some experience of the NHS, as well as running an organisation. Next there are NEDs, normally four to six; these are lay people and, if the trust is a teaching one, one NED will normally be a university representative such as the dean of the medical school. NEDs are appointed by the Secretary of State, with advice of course. Politicised commentators rail against this as another example of lack of democracy, deriding them as "ministerial stooges"[27] but in truth the NHS is an organ of a democratically elected government, so a separate democratic process for the selection of board members is not the issue, it is the ability of boards to judge and reflect the wishes and needs of the public that is the issue.

After the NEDs there are the executive members. The chief executive, medical director, the directors of nursing, of finance, and of personnel. There may be a few others, but normally these others are non-clinical senior managers, for example a chief operating officer, a director of strategy. The medical director and the director of nursing, and occasionally a dean, are the only people with any direct clinical experience on the board. The functions of executive members are clear from their titles, though they take joint responsibility for board decisions. The board as a whole essentially has five responsibilities, to:

- set the strategic direction of the organisation within the overall policies and priorities of the government and the NHS Executive
- oversee the delivery of planned results
- ensure effective financial stewardship and value for money
- ensure that high standards of corporate governance and personal behaviour are maintained
- ensure that there is effective dialogue between the organisation and the local community on its plans and performance.

Beyond that, the chairperson and non-executives have a role in the appointment, review and remuneration of the chief executive and other executive directors. Non-executive board members typically have a special interest in one or more of these areas depending on their expertise. It is hard being an NED. It is time consuming and most spend more time on it than the stipulated 20 days per year (the average is 34). It is difficult to be grafted on to an industry about which you may know little or nothing. Surveys have shown that the main activity of NEDs is simply querying and probing of executive decisions, when in theory they should be more directly involved with the strategic decision making and option appraisal. Unfortunately, NEDs tend to be quickly overloaded with the unimaginative chores of disciplinary and grievance hearings, appointment on appeal panels, and independent panels dealing with complaints. The net result is that the NHS NEDs do more than their private sector equivalents yet have difficulty focusing on the real problems in the organisation. During the last Conservative government, NEDs tended to come from commercial backgrounds and were able to come to grips with the business aspects of board activities reasonably quickly. The new government has purged 75% of these posts, the holders of which were thought to be politically unacceptable and not sensitive enough to the views of the local populace. Newer appointees are in theory made as a result of a more open process. Much was made of equality but, worryingly, the political allegiance of applicants has to be declared in advance. By 5 February 1998, 886 new NEDs had been appointed. The ethnic minority representation had been corrected, it was now 9%, which exceeded the 7% in the population as a whole. By 31 May 1998 36% of chairs and 52% of NEDs were women. Of those NEDs who said they were politically active, the overwhelming majority were Labour supporters, these included 111 Labour local councillors.

The arrangements for the new foundation hospitals as currently proposed[28] is likely to lead to some very strangely concocted boards bearing a mix of elected and unelected members with competing aspirations and very little linkage with the views that hospital staff might have as to how best they could function.[29] Whatever the future, I will guarantee that at the moment 90% of the members of staff of any trust you care to name do not know the names or the faces of their NEDs.

Much effort is put into improving the performance of boards, but many of the lists of tasks and developments needed are daunting to the point of unachievability. The anxiety is that the really talented and experienced people that the NHS needs will be put off by the unrewarding and unstimulating chores that can characterise an NED's time in the NHS.

Members of a trust board carry legal responsibilities both corporately and personally, and the Treasury Solicitor's Department has recently highlighted the adequacy of the insurance cover currently available for them so new members should check that there is appropriate insurance cover to protect them.

Clinical directors and executive groups

Boards meet on average once a month, perhaps for three hours; not long enough to manage a hospital trust, it is merely the captain's bridge. For everyday management, for the generation of new proposals, and the solution of current problems, the engine room of any trust is the executive group. This comprises the executive members of the board, that is, the chief executive, the medical director, the director of finance, etc, but to be effective it will need to draw in the next layers of the NHS hierarchy—clinical directors and non-clinical managers. How best to do this is far from certain and the solutions vary from trust to trust. The most common number of clinical directors in a trust is eight but a significant number have more than 20. In these trusts the problem is the same as throughout all organisations, how do you have an executive grouping small enough to be effective as a committee (5–15), yet not so small as to exclude the crucial range of opinion and expertise? Clinical directors can be a trifle prima donna-ish, and even downright paranoid if they feel excluded. They tend to feel that the speciality they lead is so important that it needs its own seat on the top table. But in almost all trusts there are too many of them to be in an executive group, so they need themselves to be grouped with an appointed or elected leader sitting on the executive, or else they need their own "parliament" which elects a few of its number to participate in the executive.

Whatever solution you use to bind in the clinical directors there is another problem, that of the non-clinical senior managers. So keen has the NHS been to involve doctors in management that clinical directors have been given a sort of spurious seniority in the system, they do after all have no real claim to senior management posts in that they have no special training or experience and many have no particular aptitude for it. Nor, in an egalitarian health service, do they have any moral right to be occupying most of the seats at the top table—it is an accident of history. An accident that leaves the non-clinical senior managers sometimes relegated to a major domo, adjutant, aide-de-camp or head butler role. For some no doubt that is promotion beyond their competence, but for many it is demeaning and inappropriate, so they too need to be swept up into the senior executive group. If this is not done, the danger is that they will establish a parallel network of opinion and decision taking, alongside the clinical director to chief executive axis.

The next contentious issue to be resolved is whether the chairperson of the hospital medical committee should have a seat on the executive. The members of the executive should be cabinet members sharing the decision making, so in theory there is no place for an "outsider" who may have a different agenda. The decision probably ought to be an individual one for each trust, depending on the character of the person involved.

A senior cadre

An innovative way of tying in both the clinical and non-clinical members, and others central to the working of a large organisation, is deliberately to establish a defined senior group, an officer class described in my trust with redolences of lost communism as "the senior cadre". The group meets together, debates together and is briefed together preferentially within the organisation. Senior cadre posts are graded and the grading goes with the job and with competencies, but the cadre allow egalitarian team working as all are valued equally and may, in theory, progress to any other senior cadre post. It has the added advantage of addressing the neglected problem of succession planning. A downside is that it can allow the next layer down to feel disenfranchised and can limit new blood reaching jobs that fall vacant.

References

1   Eco U. *The Name of the Rose*. London: Minerva Press, 1992, p. 218.
2   Harrison S, Hunter DJ, Pollitt C. *The Dynamics of British Health Policy*. London: Unwin Hyman, 1990, p. 2.
3   Rein M. *Social Science and Public Policy*. London: Penguin, 1976, p. 103. (Quoted by Allsop J. *Health Policy and the National Health*. London: Longman, 1984.)
4   Harrison S, Hunter DJ, Pollitt C. *The Dynamics of British Health Policy*. London: Unwin Hyman, 1990, pp 6–8.
5   Secretaries of State for Health. *Working for Patients*. Cmnd 555. London: HMSO, 1992, p. 119.
6   Department of Health (DoH). *The NHS Plan*. CM4818–1. London: The Stationery Office, 2000.
7   Butler J. *Patients, Policies and Politics*. Milton Keynes: Open University Press, 1992, p. 119.
8   Webster C. *The National Health Service, a Political History*. Oxford: Oxford University Press, 1998, p. 203.
9   Soderlund N *et al.* Impact of NHS reforms on English hospital productivity: analysis of the first three years. *BMJ* 1997;**315**:1126–9.
10 Dunleavy P, O'Leary B. *Theories of the State; the politics of liberal democracy*. London: Macmillan, 1987, pp 193–7.
11 Griffiths R (Chairman). *Report of the NHS Management Enquiry*. London: DHSS, 1983.
12 Ham C. The third way in Health care reform: does the emperor have any clothes? *J Health Services Res & Policy* 1999;**4**:168–73.
13 Eyres J, Dewar S. Delivering the NHS Plan: a case of 'constrained innovation'. In: *Health Care UK 2001*. London: King's Fund, pp 34–40.
14 Gray A, Jenkins B. Public management and the National Health Service. In: *Managing Health Care: challenges for the 90s*. London: Saunders, 1995, pp 4–32.
15 Jenkins S. *Accountable to None: the Tory nationalisation of Britain*. London: Hamish Hamilton, 1995.
16 Walshe K. The rise of regulation in the NHS. *BMJ* 2002;**324**:967–70.
17 Klein R. Governance for NHS Foundation Trusts. *BMJ* 2003;**326**:174–5.
18 Hawkes N. Comment. *The Times*, 26 July 2001, p. 18.
19 Klein R. *The Politics of the National Health Service*, 2nd edn. London: Longman, 1989.
20 Bryson B. *Notes From a Small Island*. London: Secker & Warburg, 1996.
21 Sheldon TA. Formula fever; allocating resources in the NHS. *BMJ* 1997; **315**:964.
22 Getzen TE. *Health Economics: fundamentals and flow of funds*. New York: Wiley, 1997, p. 442.
23 Klein R. *The Politics of the NHS*, 2nd edn. London: Longman, 1989.
24 Price D. Profiting from closure: the private finance initiative and the NHS. *BMJ* 1997;**315**:1479–80.
25 Pollock AM, Shaoul J, Vickers N. Private Finance and "Value for Money" in NHS hospitals: a policy in search of a rationale? *BMJ* 2002;**324**:1205–9.
26 Mitchison AA. Picture of perfection. *Sunday Telegraph Magazine* 1998; 15 February, p. 14.
27 Webster C. *The National Health Service, a Political History*. Oxford: Oxford University Press, 1998.
28 Department of Health. *A Guide to NHS Foundation Trusts*. London: DoH, 2002.
29 Klein R. Governance for NHS Foundation Trusts. *BMJ* 2003;**326**:174–5.

6: Special problems

6.1 Change

This chapter outlines some personal views about the options that clinicians or directors have in managing change. If anyone doubts the quantity and magnitude of changes engulfing the NHS in the UK, they need only weigh their non-clinical mail or review the recent year's outpouring of press releases and circulars from the Department of Health. At the time of writing there are literally dozens of "initiatives" (an Orwellian misnomer) underway with central "guidance".

Change has always been inherent in the business of medicine, but it comes in fits and starts and we are currently in the middle of a full-blown, rather protracted grand mal fit. This discomforts everyone, for it disturbs their lives and the framework that makes their lives neat and comprehensible.

Ubi stabilitas ibi religio (Where there is stability there is faith)

But without change there is no progress; though, of course, change *ipso facto* does not imply progress. The most taxing task in the business of management is the management of change, for change is the bedfellow of conflict and of stress. In dealing with the topic it is worth splitting it up into three.

1. Your personal position in relationship to change.
2. Implementing change in the organisation.
3. Responding to change by influencing upwards in the organisation.

Personal response to change

The changes that tax you most are invariably of someone else's making and their implementation may or may not be to your taste. Indeed, you would be an unimaginative and uneducated clinician if you had no views about the ideas behind any change. I suppose there are some bureaucrats who are content to act merely as a passive channel for change, a kind of crustacean effector arm. Doctors do not fit this niche in nature's hierarchy and there lies the problem for you the clinician and you the manager. Firstly, it is important to understand the medical manager's place in the process of managing change. For most clinicians caught up in the process of managing health care the changes that affect them are imposed from outside their own areas in the organisation and usually from outside the patch within which they have their regular communications and working relationships. "Outside" being government, NHS Executive, regional organisations, purchasers, Royal Colleges, and a host of other bureaucracies interested in the exercise of power without the tiresome practical difficulties of implementing their new ideas. Before you, the poor manager, try to implement someone else's bright ideas a moment's self analysis is worthwhile to review your place in "the change process". For my part I am a natural conservative, liturgically I prefer Gregorian chant and guttering candles to happy-clappy guitarists and television lights, but then that is romanticism. The chanting monk is probably tuberculous and his congregation starving, whereas happy-clappy guitarists go home in their cars to a hot lunch ...

So what is that about self analysis? Simply this. If you have an instinct to resist change think the problems through intellectually, critically read the views of others, including *BMJ* editorials, glossy government handouts, and newspaper comment, and decide whether you are wholeheartedly in support of change or at least acquiescent towards it. Conversely, if you find the business of change stimulating and the rollercoaster of making it happen exciting, look into your soul—or rather your physiology—to check that you are not just getting a buzz from the adrenaline. That done, old reactionaries or young revolutionaries may place themselves in relation to change. If they disagree with it for good objective reasons that they can support in debate then they should object in the right forum. If they still object after the debate they should resign or swallow their pride and do the best they can to implement the change without spending time denying its value to all and sundry.

That is all very simple, reality is usually more difficult. Take, for example, the easygoing timetable that many junior doctors enjoy consequent upon the implementation of the EWTD (European Working Time Directive). Many of us feel deeply

Figure 6.1 Responses to change.

unhappy about it for reasons we can argue; it erodes the vocational thread that should imbue a career in medicine, and in practical terms it can interfere with the continuity of patient care and the education of young doctors. But it is the law (even European law is law). Most junior doctors want it and perhaps the drawbacks may be overcome; so let us support it while trying to ameliorate the problems it generates.

The response of individuals and groups to change usually follows this pattern (Figure 6.1).

Although your self respect will demand that you continue to comment *upwards* (*see below*) and at executive level on changes you think inappropriate, you must be consistent when working towards achieving them. This is not simply a matter of cabinet responsibility, it is a practical matter of being credible as a manager. Effective implementation does not mean you have to deny problems. It is a matter of how you do it and the most important thing is that whoever you are leading should not be confused by your actions, wondering if you really want them to implement the change or not.

Implementing change

Nothing would ever be attempted if all possible objections must first be overcome

(Sam Johnson)

The actual process of planning change needs to be handled in a cool, sequential way. There will be plenty of room for gesture and intuition in the day-to-day hurly burly of implementation. The important first step is a careful overview to ensure the following.

- *Define the change and prioritise it* among other changes that are planned.
- *Identify the effects the change will have* on people, on the organisation as a whole, and on the functions of its departments. Make sure you know all the ramifications of the change you propose. How many people and actions will this change affect? Did you realise that moving ENT from one hospital to another affects the day-to-day management of stroke victims because the speech therapy department will need to move too? Did you know that removing children's services from one hospital to another may lose your anaesthetic department its educational recognition? Now revisit the change and decide if you still want to make it. If you do, make a preliminary assessment of the steps needed to achieve the change. This must be done in consultation with those who will be affected.
- If having looked at the details you still plan to go ahead, *communicate the changes* openly, honestly, and widely— remembering that those who oppose change often do so late and affect not to have been told about it earlier. Consultants, in particular, sometimes give the impression

that if they have not been informed verbally and personally they could not be expected to know about change. Some major changes require formal public consultation especially if services are to be removed from one hospital to another. This is a time consuming and difficult process and will need to be orchestrated by an outside agency, usually the local purchasing authority.

- *Do not overstate or misrepresent* the benefits of the change you plan. Audiences are sophisticated about the implications of change; indeed, they might be more sophisticated than you.
- *Reappraise the project* yet again in the light of the feedback you have had from the communication exercise. This is particularly important because there are often knock-on effects from change, which are not immediately apparent or are minimised by the enthusiasts who want the change. Very few changes are universally welcomed; thus the difficult part of the process is often to hold firm where there are a large number of opponents yet the bulk of the evidence suggests that the change is necessary and beneficial.

Once you have clearly embarked on the process of change opponents may start to use alternative channels to prevent it. They will appeal over your head to more senior people within the organisation. They will appeal outside the organisation. They will try to sway those who previously supported the change, and if they feel passionately about it they will not be beyond dirty tricks, misinformation, and disinformation; hence the importance of the next phase.

- *Commitment planning*: the neat concept described by Barnes[1] requires an analysis of who in the organisation needs to be committed to the change, what role they need to play, where they stand now, and how they need to change if things are to happen smoothly. Barnes identified four categories of commitment for key participants:

    "*No Commitment*"—likely to oppose the change.
    "*Let It Happen*"—will not oppose the initiative but will not actively support it.
    "*Help It Happen*"—must provide resources (time or equipment).
    "*Make It Happen*"—must be actively involved and willing to lead.

Key players	No commitment	Let it happen	Help it happen	Make it happen
Chief executive officer				OX
Chairman St Judes medical staff committee	O ⟶	X		
UMB member A		O ⟶		X
UMB member B			O ⟶	X
Consultant C		O ⟶ X		
Consultant D		X ⟵		O
Manager E		O ⟶		X

O = present position; X = required position.
(Consultant D has poor interpersonal skills and his enthusiasm is likely to be counterproductive)

Figure 6.2 Charting personal commitment to change. (Reproduced with permission from: Simpson and Smith, *Management for Doctors*. London: BMJ Books, 1995.)

He suggests that this exercise is done formally and the positions of key participants tabulated (Figure 6.2).

- *Action planning*: having gathered all views on the original proposal, sifted them, rejected some, and incorporated some, it is time formally to list all the actions needed to reach the goal. Some of these will be on the critical path, that is, if they do not happen or do not happen on time everything else is delayed. In most projects it helps to construct a Gantt chart (Figure 6.3). This is easy for most of those involved to understand and helps to focus everyone's minds on the "choke points" in the implementation process.

I have carefully not called this stage the "business planning stage", though the elements of a business plan will need to be there identifying the targets, the route, the resources to be used, the cost, and the benefits versus the disadvantages. However, too formal a business planning process has in my experience a deadening, even stupefying effect and may be totally counterproductive if teams are expected to produce a watertight, polished plan relating to something fluid and evolving.

It is, however, critical at this stage to identify which staff will be involved in making change happen and whether extra resources are needed. Taking staff away from their normal roles can be disruptive, and the ill effects of this are quickly used by detractors further to pillory the process and those involved. Having identified staff it is important to identify a *project manager* even for a small project who can be set a target and timetable.

- *Reappraisal*: having followed through the above steps, revisit the concept that set the change process in motion. Does it still make sense? Can you still afford it? Will it achieve what you want? Detailed, honest planning often shows up a need for more personnel and resources than you had at first thought, so decide if you still wish to go ahead or whether you could better put the effort to something else on your list of priorities. To conclude that it is "too much hassle for too little gain" is a perfectly honourable conclusion and not going ahead is not necessarily a sign of managerial weakness.
- *Recommunicate*: yes, we are going ahead and here is the plan.
- *Go for it!* Projects that limp along slowly demoralise everyone. Money, staff, and enthusiasm leach away into more achievable ends and managerial credibility is lost.

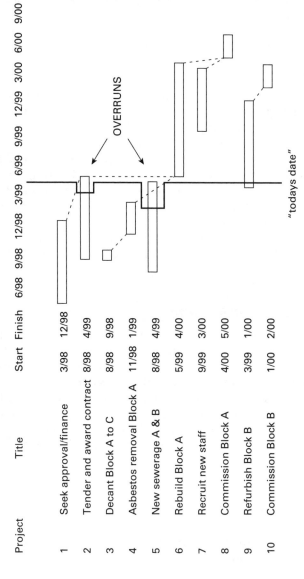

Figure 6.3 A Gantt chart.

Delaying because of quibbles over cost is common. Quibbles about small, overbudget items tend to be counterproductive because the delay and extra work that is incurred have a habit of costing more than the quibble would have saved.

During implementation keep the team informed, especially about problems. One of the most successful projects I have watched underway carried everyone along with it because the architect's drawings were attached to the walls, the work could be seen progressing, the stage in the timetable, and the problems with the project were all honestly and briefly annotated and stuck up as wall posters from day to day.

Lastly, do not forget that the completion of a change project, whether it be new procedures, a new building or the start-up of a new service, requires major commitment to *training and induction* for all those involved. Too often neither budget nor time are set aside for this.

When the project is complete and successful *announce it, be proud about it,* and make sure you thank all those whose hard work might otherwise go unrecognised.

Managing responses upwards

"Managing up" is the business of influencing the organisational levels above you so as to modulate if necessary the projects they are asking you to implement. It covers everything from a response to a draft proposal from government to a frank workers' revolt. It is an important concept because the notion that "managing up" can and does occur goes a long way to alleviate the sense of powerlessness that so many in the NHS feel. Given the enormous size of the NHS and the great distance between central decision makers and the health service coalface, you would think that as a medical manager your options for influencing policy retroactively are small. This is not so. Regardless of the shifts towards deprofessionalisation and marginalisation of doctors that has occurred, they still nonetheless have the moral whiphand in most situations, and if they are honest and careful they can still be regarded as the arbiters of what is appropriate in health care.

The ways for doctors to "manage up" are multitudinous; some are proper and some are improper. As a clinician you can manage up by way of the BMA and its representatives or the Royal Colleges and their representatives. They both have ways into the decision-making processes. If you are a manager you can and should join BAMM (the British Association of Medical Managers), and if you are a medical director, the Association of Trust Medical Directors. Occasionally you will have a chance to express a view to visiting inspection teams, such as those from CHAI, visiting dignitaries, chairs of health boards, MPs, junior ministers. If you really feel that is likely to be a useful channel you should carefully orchestrate your approach in advance and decide who says what and when. Passionate gripes over coffee are ill received; quiet exposure to the practical aspects of the problem during the tour is more likely to be effective. A "memory bite" to match the politician's "sound bite".

The problem about professional organisations as formal channels for "managing up" when change is afoot is that, although government "initiatives" are sent out for consultation, the timescale for these "consultation exercises" is, either through incompetence or design, so short as to make a considered view difficult and a properly researched one impossible. The BMA is often given only a few weeks in which to reply, whereas those of us further down the line will often receive our papers after the date for receipt of replies. So, unsurprisingly, other ways of being heard are forced upon us.

Your next weapon is formal letters to policymakers, solicited or unsolicited. These need careful handling. Non-clinical managers are always amazed at doctors' preference for writing letters rather than making face-to-face contact but that is the way we do things and in many contexts the good letter is effective. The angry/outraged/passionate letter is all very well but remember always:

- sleep on what you have written before sending it
- share it with another person before you send it
- get your facts right!

Even if your letter is nine-tenths right it will be tarnished by wrong facts or assumptions. Even a wrong paragraph will tarnish a whole letter and allow the minister's aide with a smile to fold it neatly into a paper dart and launch it at the wastepaper basket.

Oh, and by the way, don't send out too many copies. I have seen letters of the most trivial nature copied to the Prime Minister, the Secretary of State, the presidents of all the Royal Colleges, etc, etc. By all means copy but try to pick the people who are likely to see it and whose actions are genuinely likely to be changed by your letter.

Next, the most dangerous option of all, the media.

The media

I mention this here to dismiss it as a proper means of "managing up". It is useful to believe that the press is a whore, pretending to please but intent only on its own profit. The information it uses is usually unvalidated, biased, and inconsistent; its use of that information cynical. At the top of the broadsheet tree it makes some efforts to be responsible (though less effort to be accurate) and at the bottom of the tabloid tree it makes efforts only to amaze, alarm, titivate or amuse. Your own attempts at forcing change on an unwilling government or disgruntled doctors' attempts to change the plans your trust has carefully construed are all grist to the mill when seen from the press's point of view. They will believe what you tell them, flatter, and cajole you into saying more than you should, and in a day they will be gone, your passionate concerns turned into chip wrappings. All personal relations with the media risk bringing out your worst streaks of vanity, and appearance on the television verges on reckless self exposure as all your normal reflexes towards caution and balance are abandoned.

It is not all true of course but if you believe that it is almost true it may help you to keep out of trouble. If you must deal with the media do so through or with the advice of a professional public relations officer. If having to deal with the media is a habit then go on a course to learn how to do it safely.

Types of change

The sort of changes that will affect you may be categorised in five ways.

1. *Ideological change*: political change, imposition of performance targets, the establishment of primary care trusts.

2. *Legislative change*: changes in employment legislation.
3. *Functional change*: the managerial meat, for example service reconfigurations, mergers, enlarging, shrinking, etc.
4. *Technical change*: owing to advances in medical care, for example setting up non-invasive surgery.
5. *Fatuous change*: these changes may not in themselves be inappropriate or harmful but are those embarked on for cosmetic or fashion reasons, for example changing the logo on the notepaper.

Another categorisation of change is simply to divide it into big projects and little projects. Big projects, such as working time directives or reducing junior doctors' hours, are those where the endpoint is defined but the mechanics of getting there are not always clear, and the funding almost invariably absent. It is these sort of projects that have the greater power to demotivate and demoralise teams. Little projects, by contrast, if well done and funded tend to be achievable and achieved, and give all those involved a sense of satisfaction. Small is beautiful.

Incremental change and large projects

Because of the difficulties of large projects their achievement needs to be divided up very carefully into bite-sized pieces at the outset. In particular, this involves setting realistic targets. One of the most irritating features of the government's pet projects is the frequent assumption that everything can be achieved within a very short timespan. This is often impossible for managers and leads merely to confrontation between visiting enforcement teams and managers who have not achieved targets, and between managers who are not achieving and clinicians who cannot deliver the service if the changes were imposed quickly with inadequate resources. New managers have a habit of wanting the shiny, full-built end product quickly and may need to be reminded that this is not always the appropriate way forward. One new postgraduate dean had to be taken aside and told "You have too many objectives that require explicit action". That sounds Byzantine but was at least pragmatic. The same postgraduate dean told me that dealing with the almost unachievable big projects that were required of him was like banging his head against jelly; all the frustrations but none of the relieving pleasure of pain that he would have had if it had been a wall.

Small change projects

People will commit an enormous amount of effort to small local projects, an extension to a ward, a new ITU, a refurbished clinic, a new piece of technology, a new way of running a clinic, a new way of delivering education. As a medical manager or member of an executive group, you will be brought many of these proposals and your wish to be positive and supportive needs to be tempered by some practicalities. You might usefully ask the following questions of the project.

- Is it really needed?
- Is it thought through?
- Is it properly costed?
- Are the knock-on effects on other specialities or areas understood?
- Will it fly? That is, can it be funded?
- Does it rely on the enthusiasm of only one person?
- Is there space?
- What will happen down the line one to five years from now?
- How does it fit in with the institution's overall needs and plans?
- Is it the most appropriate thing on which to expend your energies?

As a medical manager or member of a committee you have useful experience that may be brought to bear on the critical appraisal of such proposals. You can protect the organisation from:

- zany ideas
- overbidding
- shroud waving
- undeclared effects on other departments.

After a while you become sensitive to the ploys which enthusiastic, well-meaning clinicians bring to bear on the presentation of their pet projects. Standard bidding ploys include the following.

- "It will bring in extra money." (*Your response*: "Prove it, is the money out there?")
- "If we don't have it we will not be recognised as a serious unit/by the SAC/for university training." (*Your response*: "Who said so? When was a unit last derecognised for not having this?")
- "If we don't have it patients will suffer." (*Your response*: "How? Prove it!")
- "If we don't have it we cannot recruit/retain staff." (*Your response*: "What is your current staff turnover? What evidence do you have that the absence of this is losing you staff?")

Of course you must not just baldly recite this killjoy's catechism, your normal tone will naturally be positive and encouraging, avoiding the traditional "The answer's 'No!' now what's the question?"

Project overload

For the upper echelons of management there is a tendency to commission or embrace more and more projects. Being positive about the NHS seems to dictate it and not to respond implies that you are unaware of the "climate of change" and indeed that if you are not responding you are not managing in all senses of the word; so the upper echelons of management have a reprehensible habit of passing on all these initiatives half digested to the middle and lower grade managers and their clinical colleagues. And why not? The cynic would say that the initiators do not have to do the work, the middle managers who work through the project do not mind, if they did their *raison d'être* would evaporate anyway why would they because the chores, the leg work requires effort not by them but by subcommittees, doctors, nurses, physiotherapists, secretaries, and others further down in the organisation, so what is the problem? The problem is one of overload.

Overload is tolerated by the workers when it is judged to be appropriate. Doctors and nurses will work tirelessly when patients' needs are the imperative. Junior managers will work to open a ward or deal with a backlog, but when a project is not understood or not agreed upon by the "doers" it will not happen. This is a major problem in the NHS where so many "initiatives" are seen as superfluous to the core business of health care. The argument that the latest initiative is just to tidy up the remaining loose ends does not ring true either. The "last push" is seen by most clinicians in the same light as a subaltern's in the first world war ordered to make "the final push", rather than the midwife urging a final push when all but the baby's legs are in view. How do we control the flow of projects? Essentially, it is a matter of "managing up", as described earlier, something of which boards, executives, and senior managers do too little and to which the NHS Executive, regions, and colleges are too impervious. It would be nice if there were coupons or some form of rationing for the DoH and the NHS Executive. If they were only allowed five new initiatives a year they might think through the ones they proposed a little more carefully and spend more time on less projects, rather than inadequate time on a large number. The NHS Executive, in common with all other layers of senior management should always consider before starting a new initiative whether or not the managerial effort might not be better spent in ensuring that the last project commissioned had actually been implemented and was having the intended effect. Senior managers in the NHS intent on radical change might usefully read Hobsbawm on the French Revolution. He observed that it succeeded because the changes were formalised by philosophers into an intellectually coherent set of plans, and were effective because they genuinely reflected the people's needs. The people could focus on the reasons for their dissent and could understand and support each solution at a personal level, whether it was land reform, reduced taxation, fair local administration, or whatever. So many of the changes forced on to the NHS fail because they have not been formalised in an intellectually or economically credible way and are couched in such terms that the ordinary peasants working in the health service have difficulty perceiving them to be of personal relevance.

6.2 Rationalisations and mergers

It is less than 10 years since the government of the day thought that merger and shrinkage of units was the best way to achieve clinical and cost efficiency. As ever, "experts" were on hand to "prove" that less beds were needed and that more and more day case care and shorter and shorter lengths of stay were readily achievable. It is less than five years since the government woke up to the disasterous consequences of these policies and the pressure to merge units as a way of reducing beds has largely passed. But, the UK is still bedevilled by too many small units and the need for a smaller number of centres each filled with expert staff working no more than 48 hours a week continues to revivify the habit of merger and rationalisation.

The stress of mergers

It is a fact of life that Nature is red in tooth and claw, and large animals eat smaller ones. So with mergers. The naturally predatory behaviour of all organisations leads them to enjoy colonisations, which sounds unkind but is true. Nine times out of 10 there are winners, and winners enjoy being winners, and of course losers hate being losers; all of this generates a lot of angst but does not slow the process too much. Mergers where the two parties are of equal sizes carry the most difficulties. For example, the merger of Guy's and St Thomas' hospitals in London was agonisingly difficult. Both hospitals were of the same size, same budget, same fame (each, of course, would dispute that), and had the same sized power base, but they were culturally different. The decision as to the dominant partner in a geographical sense was decided on data that could (but not necessarily should) have been argued to the opposite conclusion. In fact, there was no very obvious winner and loser, both organisations won something and both lost something; but Guy's perceived itself the loser and the delicacy of the equation goaded many people working within the organisation to subvert the process of merger in large or small ways. Whether that was an admirable commitment to a different vision or just short-sighted cussedness is a matter of opinion, but it certainly helped no one in the long term except some politicians. The situation in other mergers is, I am told, similar.

Could these, or any other mergers, have been managed differently? Looking back the answer is almost certainly a grudging "Yes". A shorter timescale for the decision, a definite timescale for the grieving, and then much more forceful efforts to get on with normal life would undoubtedly improve the process for the participants. Doctors who spend their lives dealing with mortal illness ought to know about these things. However, I confess that it was only in the midst of the Guy's and St Thomas' merger that I came to realise how like a death it seemed for many at Guy's, how important is the management of grieving, and how important it is to understand that the behaviour of some was akin to that of those close to a dying person: inappropriately focused anger, denial, and inability to function effectively.

The arrangement of a merger between departments or hospitals taps into some of the deepest human feelings. Feelings about sacred places, tribal kinship, hierarchical status, and the responsibilities of a continuous lineage. These are feelings familiar and fascinating to the social anthropologist but a major problem for managers; so the first and crucial message about merger is to be very sensitive to those feelings, be very wary of the trouble they will cause, and be very, very sure of the benefits that might accrue from merger. Has the team's morale been valued sufficiently? Will the benefits of merger be sufficient to justify the problems you are about to cause yourself and others? Which leads to the second message, that is, do not expect all the planned benefits of a merger actually to accrue. A certain overstatement of the benefits is necessary to energise the people involved but do not fool yourself that they will happen. Assumptions about the financial benefits of merger which have been well documented as being false both in the USA and the UK. It is against this background that managers should plan mergers. Non-clinical managers rarely understand the *volksgeist*, the cultural pride of the clinical teams involved, a feeling that may have built up over many years and have been reinforced by the clonal selection processes of generations of interview committees. When teams of different cultures are merged, a lot of problems appear which would not have been predicted. Every little thing can cause trouble:

"We do it like this."
"Oh well, I am sorry but we do it like this."

Some people may make much of these differences further to discredit the merger. In other businesses and in industry, you simply get rid of people who are inappropriately obstructing a process that the organisation knows must happen, but in the NHS you normally have to keep them in post, and it may be years before their negative effect works its way out of the system. It has been said that corporate mergers take 10 years to settle down and have everybody working for the common goal. I suspect that is an underestimate. One of the added problems is that the NHS has no established arbitration process for resolving merger issues, the prelude to mergers can therefore become even more acrimonious than it might, with long-term ill effects.[2]

One might reasonably think the common goal is the care of patients. Sad to say, the tribal reflexes of groups in the NHS seeking to preserve their identity, their traditions, and their original territories will all too often overwhelm that basic principle. Lack of enthusiasm for mergers is not solely the province of doctors and patients as is sometimes claimed. A survey of 500 senior NHS managers, by the Institute of Health Services Management, found that "one out of every three managers believed that the drive for mergers was purely politically motivated and 93% believed them to be disruptive, 73% disagreed with NHS research that claimed that hospitals with less than 300 beds are uneconomic." Hardly the responses one would hope to see in the group central to the implementation of mergers but this is not surprising. Doctors and nurses rarely lose their jobs during mergers, managers do—and even if they do not they may have to weather an uncomfortable period when there is uncertainty about their future, they may have to apply for their own jobs in the new joint organisation. It is hardly surprising therefore that unless the futures of at least the senior management team are settled right at the beginning of a merger process, the very people who need to make it happen will be less than fully committed to the task.

All in all it must be best to avoid mergers if possible, as they can fuel instability and anxiety, cause major disruption, need huge amounts of managerial support,[3] and rarely achieve their objectives. "It is not at all clear from the evidence whether such marriages are 'made in heaven' or are simply politically convenient as a perceived 'quick fix' which ultimately deflects attention from difficult choices about Health Care priorities".[4] Even citing quality gain as a justification for mergers is difficult to substantiate from published evidence. In the USA, where efficiency gains are cited as evidence that a merger is necessary, some proposed mergers have been challenged in court which usually found the cases unpersuasive on the evidence offered.

There are some basic principles which could help mergers work, but they seem only rarely to be applied:

- do very, very careful research to determine whether merger is really necessary
- involve all the key participants early
- define the plan and stick to it
- make senior appointments to the new merged unit early and with a minimum duration of uncertainty
- communicate, communicate, communicate
- FUND IT ADEQUATELY.

6.3 Rationing

Of course rationing of health care exists, it always did, and always will, and the recent promises of extra cash for the NHS will not vitiate it. The problem with rationing in the NHS is that the current systems for rationing are "inefficient, inequitable, undemocratic and opaque".[5] Anyone who works within the NHS knows this to be the case and knows how subtle rationing can be. For example, the old lady who does not call her GP because she considers him to be too busy. The GP who does not refer her to hospital with her renal failure because he believes that limited resources should not be used to dialyse old ladies in renal failure; the unwillingness to order a test for her because the waiting list for such tests is too long. The inability for her to see a nephrologist because nephrologists are in such short supply and so on. We have all lived with this state of affairs for many years, but doctors, managers, and particularly doctor-managers become more frustrated by it as the pressures to ration increase and an increasing openness in society makes it inescapable that one must admit that it is happening and explain why. This state of affairs is made worse by consecutive governments, none of which has had the courage to admit the reality of the situation, who have twisted and turned, and talked as if the managerial revolution or efficiency or prioritisation or mergers or the private finance initiative, or even when all that fails, a little more cash will solve the problem but have never, ever mentioned the "R word". In 1994, Duncan Nichol who had been chief executive of the NHS and presumably could have been expected to understand how the NHS worked, established a group to stimulate debate about the future of the NHS and rationing, and to clarify policy. That group concluded, not unreasonably, that rationing would be necessary. Yet Stephen Dorrell, the Secretary of State at that time, inappropriately quoting HL Mencken, said Nichol's group's analysis was "simple, obvious and wrong".

Demand for health care and new options for providing health care expand faster than provision and, whatever government ministers may say, sooner or later explicit rationing will have to come into play. I have a thick file crammed with papers and comment saying just this. Some date back many years yet none of them announces a realistic government-driven initiative to explore a common national framework in which limited health resources can be used efficiently and equitably. The British habit of "muddling through" appears to be the officially sanctioned policy. NICE, one could argue, is just a sophisticated, well-intentioned way of trying to be fair and rational while evading the "R word". This does not mean there is not action, and indeed some of the actions are driven by central government, but they are few and none of the actions have led to a structure whereby clinical managers have a consistent set of administrative rules by which they respond to inadequate provision. That responsibility has been devolved to separate health authorities and to a plethora of different sticking plaster remedies, the only point of this process being that the health authority outside the hospital and managers inside the hospital are demonised as the agents of rationing. Since there is no central acknowledgement of the need to ration, any rationing that actually occurs is perceived as a fault of hospitals, a dereliction of duty by managers, or bloody mindedness by doctors. There is no immediate end to this in sight, so to help medical managers understand why they will remain in the mire, the remainder of this section deals with current means by which resource use is restrained and then offers a discussion on some of the areas that medical managers' successors will need to watch in the future.

Current mechanisms of rationing

The primary agent in rationing is the fixed budget. This, in subtle or unsubtle format, works from the top of the NHS to the bottom. The rationing of surgical care by waiting list is perhaps the clearest example; the inability to afford beds and operating time leads to a waiting list. It does indeed force an increase in day surgery and shorter stays but these do not suffice and the waiting list remains in place. Health authorities could and regularly do earmark more money to reduce the waiting list if they judge the operations present on the waiting list to be of sufficient clinical importance and the regular panic event of the "waiting list initiative" shows what can be achieved, but in most prioritisation exercises the treatment of low urgency surgical problems does not score highly. Health purchasing authorities may simply ration by allocating an inadequate global budget, but in most instances they now attempt to be more proactive and specify how their finite budget is to be used by providers of care. In making that sort of judgment the issues are normally considered extremely carefully in a multidisciplinary debate informed by judgments about efficacy and importance, and the needs of the specific population that the purchaser serves. But, however carefully the exercise is carried out there will always be patients left outside; that is what rationing is about. You can fudge the issue by not being too explicit and by not insisting that a decision should cover everyone in the population but all that does is push the decision-making process back to where it always was—with clinicians. In the meantime, all that has happened is that excluded patients become angry. This can happen even in apparently non-contentious decisions. Lewisham, Southwark, and Lambeth Health Authority was once threatened with judicial review by HIV organisations after removing complementary medicine and osteopathy from a list of interventions it was willing to purchase! Explicit decisions tend to be at the margins, as Klein observes: "the price of visibility is triviality".[6] Even so lack of central support for the principle of exclusion means that even where you have a policy that excludes the excision of sebaceous cysts and tattoos, doctors are left having to argue with patients or managers to argue with clinicians. If the sebaceous cyst not worthy of operation turns out to be a bizarre and atypical sarcoma then God help you; the lawyers and your trust will not.

The much-reported case of Jamie B is an example of attempts at rationing by an individual health authority being unsupported. Cambridgeshire and Huntingdon Health Authority made what it believed to be a good moral and clinical case for not funding yet more chemotherapy for this child with terminal leukaemia, but the patient's relatives and the media thought otherwise and the unfortunate and unsupported health authority became victims of the lack of clarity about how rationing decisions should be made. The chief executive's reflections on the case make instructive reading. His conclusions reflecting on the experience were that:

> Making decisions on issues of such profound importance to citizens, is a matter for government, indeed a matter for national debate and resolution.
>
> The quality of the process by which decisions are arrived at is as important as the actual outcomes. The process requires explicit documèntation of clinical evidence, self-confidence, compassion and a preparedness to communicate these widely.[7]

However, it is always going to be difficult for a bureaucratic organisation, primarily perceived as dealing in cash rather than patients, to make difficult decisions. In theory, it may be easier for primary care trusts to deny treatment. Nevertheless, this has the moral difficulty of putting doctors in the invidious position of making financially based judgments about rationing that might be different from their clinical judgments. That is what we have all been doing for many years. What is different now is that we are expected to be open about it and thus are abused for it. This is the nub of the problem. Whatever the gymnastics that have preceded a decision to limit access to treatment, the final decision is properly and normally made by clinicians and is thus properly a repeated exercise in clinical judgment, not just an exercise in policing lists drawn up by health authorities. Whereas allocation decisions were made privately and quietly in good faith in the past, they may now only be sustained when made openly, honestly, and in public if individual clinicians' decisions are set against a national rationing framework that has been properly debated and publicly accepted and that admits a need for doctors to make decisions about allocation.

So where do medical managers go from here? Firstly, they need to keep an eye on the debate. At the moment, because the government does not engage in it, the debate is akin to Dutch Protestants planning the future of the Church of Rome, but perhaps things will change. Secondly, the debate as published is likely to be confusing, diffuse, and circular to the average reader. I challenge anyone to get any sense of satisfaction or any perception of progress out of a review of the last five years' articles on rationing in the *British Medical Journal*.

The future of rationing: steps to watch

A better decision-taking process

By the creation of NICE (the National Institute of Clinical Excellence) the government took a major step towards establishing a mechanism that might address perceived and real failures in access to useful healthcare interventions. Because of the limited scope of NICE's recommendations, and because the evidence shows that its advice is often ignored by local purchasers, a better and agreed process for decision taking at local level needs to be established when central government does not take these decisions (the removal of dental services and eye tests, the closure of psychiatric institutions, and the limiting of breast screening to women aged under 65 are, it should be remembered, central rationing decisions). Local processes will need to be very open, very well informed by an evidence base that looks not just at outcome in a life expectancy sense but also more at quality. Nevertheless, on balance, most opinion seems to support the necessity of central decision making about major rationing issues so as to avoid the "rationing by postcode" which occurs when different health authorities make different decisions. NICE exists as the mechanism which might assist in these processes but like all regulatory bodies it needs to show itself to be competent, independent, and powerful enough to have its recommendations accepted by government without any deliberating. NICE, however, only addresses the detail of what is provided, not the global issues of what the NHS can realistically afford to do in the long term.

A more intelligent national debate

There is a need for a more intelligent national debate on what core services the NHS should supply. What mechanism should be used to decide what is in the core?[8] New Zealand, Norway, Oregon, and Holland have all famously addressed these issues, none with satisfactory outcomes, and none in a similar way. Oregon established a prioritised list of treatments and funded the best 565 of 696 options. Holland refined the process by which decisions would be made and identified effectiveness and efficiency as crucial limiters, but like everyone else simply ended up rationing services such as homoeopathy and adult dental care (Figure 6.4). However, both Holland and New Zealand rejected the excluding nature of the Oregon exercise and fixed on the establishment of guidelines for clinical care based on consensus conferences. The basic tenet is "only provide what works". All these exercises involved the public in the debate. The British government seems to prefer to move in the direction of the New Zealand initiative with the stress on guidelines, hoping somehow to restrict treatment that a formal evaluation process (NICE) does not find "clinically effective". The French have established an equivalent organisation, ANAES (Agence Nationale d'Accréditation et d'Evaluation en Santé)—like NICE acronymically reassuring if worryingly Orwellian.

Involvement of the public

A lot of lip service is attached to the need to involve the public, but how to involve them in a meaningful rather than token way is more difficult. Focus groups are fashionable but of course undemocratic; conferences with lay participation similarly. It is, however, known that the public is prepared to display altruism and understand that some members may have to forego some care to allow the proper treatment of sicker others. Additionally, the public is known to be unhappy about local rather than national processes being used for rationing. Lastly, the public does expect to be involved.[9] When it is involved its priorities differ somewhat from those of GPs and of consultants, but not hugely.[10] The exact process by which the public may declare its preferences for health care might start from a proposal made by Ronald Dworkin, an American professor of law and a medical ethicist. Professor Dworkin proposed that the public should be asked to imagine a world with five characteristics.

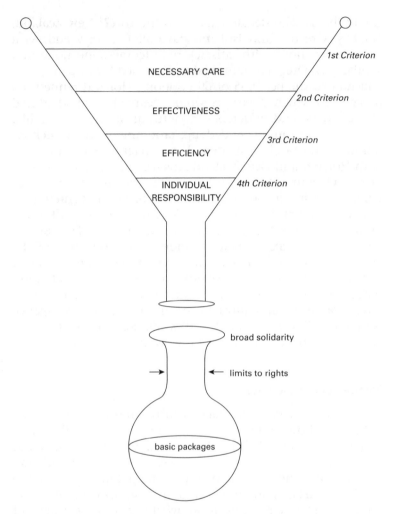

Figure 6.4 The conceptual framework proposed by the Dunning
Committee to determine healthcare priorities. The much quoted
"Dunning Filter" filtered out much the same avoidable care as others
have proposed: adult dental care, homoeopathic medicine, etc.

1. That everybody has the same amount of money to spend.
2. That information about medicine and its effectiveness is
   accurate and freely available.
3. That everybody's interests, children, adults and the
   elderly, are put at the same level.

4.   That everyone is assumed to be at the same risk of disease.
5.   That people make decisions rationally.

In this imaginary world people would need to buy an imaginary insurance policy but would have to specify what was to be covered by that policy. Professor Dworkin argued that, for example, few would buy a health insurance policy that offered them lifesaving treatment if they fell into a persistent vegetative state, nor did he think that there would be many takers for a policy that offered lifesaving treatment in the late stages of dementia and so on. A number of interventions currently regularly provided would quickly be excluded. His predictions may or may not be true but the idealistic scenario which he presents illustrates an academically reasonable starting point for a debate.[11] If the public is to be involved the media will play a large part in influencing its views. At the moment the media is so immature and sensationalist in its attitude to the health issue that it could be dangerously counterproductive to involve it.

Realistically, public debate may do a little to control demand and will not increase supply unless it acquiesces to tax increases but it might help increase the acceptability of gaps between supply and demand and the practical mechanics of administering rationing. The sceptic will nevertheless point out that the public as a healthy generality, and the patient as a sick specific, differ widely in their opinions. The public as a whole is very likely to say that the millions earmarked for the use of beta interferon for MS (multiple sclerosis), a remitting disease might be better spent elsewhere. The MS Society and patients with an acute exacerbation of their MS might disagree. What this points to is the problem of who shall be the responsible agent for taking the recommendations of NICE or of citizen's juries and enforcing them in the clinic?

A radical rethink about how the NHS delivers care

This seems the unlikely horse at the back of the field, carrying too heavy an ideological burden to give it a chance of winning, but you never know. If it does put in a showing perhaps it will be along the lines of the NHS contracting to provide only truly core services and requiring individuals to insure themselves if they want the remainder. Weale pointed out that in a world of limited resources we have to resolve an *inconsistent triad*, "a collection of propositions any two of which are compatible with each other but which when viewed together in a threesome form a contradiction".[12] He implies that we can have one of the three possible pairs in the triad of comprehensiveness, quality and availability. We can have either:

- a comprehensive service of high quality but not available to all (as in the USA)
- a comprehensive service freely available to all but not of high quality (the NHS)
- a high-quality service freely available to all but not comprehensive (that is, excellent core coverage but no more).

New technology assessment

Technology is the military arm of science, it articulates our preference for action over inaction and adsorbs our obsession with the new. It is also expensive and often harmful. Even if the current allocation for health care were sufficient and there was no rationing, one could be fairly certain that the advent of new technologies and new drugs, new high-cost procedures, or new low-cost high-volume procedures would upset the applecart in the future. The problem at the moment is that these new arrivals can take root at hospital level with minimal control, usually without a formal business plan or consultation with purchasers, even without consultation with other groups within the hospital such as a prescribing committee, a clinical director, or the director of finance who might have a view. The new technology simply insinuates itself and provides a constant pressure on resources. If we were able to control these new technologies and use the ones which were truly valuable, and were able to make a judgment about them *before* they began to be implemented widely in hospitals we might have a humane rationing weapon. There are many examples of widespread inappropriate and expensive use of new technology before its assessment. For example, laparoscopic repair of inguinal hernias. Inguinal hernias can, of course, normally be repaired as a day case under local anaesthetic with minimal discomfort and an early return to work. Laparoscopic hernia repairs require a general anaesthetic, an invasion of the abdominal cavity, the use of disposable instruments whose cost exceeds the current total cost of an outpatient hernia operation; and all this to produce an operation whose only benefit in a first-time unilateral hernia is possibly to return the patients to work a day or so earlier. Two cunningly juxtaposed articles in the *BMJ* of 4th May 2002 neatly illustrated the problem. One, by Motson, argued that NICE should have approved laparoscopic hernia repair but underplayed the potential severity of complications and neglected to mention the advances in open repair done as a day case under local anaesthetic. He is an enthusiast, of course, for laparoscopic repair. The adjacent paper[13] reviewed the lessons to be learnt in retrospect from the use of "supralethal" chemotherapy with marrow transplantation; initially hailed by its enthusiasts as the best form of chemotherapy for breast cancer and supported in the USA by special interest groups of such vociferousness that women took to court insurance companies who would not fund it. Calm, independent assessment eventually showed it to be no better yet certainly more risky than cheaper, kinder forms of chemotherapy. A chilling paper well worth reading. The drive for the use of new technology is too often simply clinicians looking for novelty (kindly called *innovators*), pressure from instrument companies, clinicians wishing not to be left behind, and sometimes possibly hospitals wishing to show that they are doing "up-to-date" things. If new technology assessment as a form of rationing is to take root, much more mature media reporting is going to be needed. At present the media is perfectly prepared to report enthusiastically on totally spurious, unvalidated alternative therapies for cancer, etc, so one wonders how it might respond to limitation of a slightly effective but very expensive treatment which is to be withheld.

Demand management

This concerns education and access to information as much as anything. The use of telephone helplines like NHS Direct, for example, may be shown to reduce callouts of doctors and attendances at accident and emergency departments but not by much. Better education might reduce the expectation that to be effective the GP needs to prescribe something or to refer to a hospital.[14]

The practicalities

Much of what is written on rationing is academic and fixes on the "what" not the "how". For the foreseeable future medical managers will be the bouncers at the door as far as rationing is concerned. There is no prospect of this task becoming any easier so what advice can they be given?

- If there are explicit restrictions make sure they are in writing and that you know who they came from and the process by which they were established.
- Make sure that restrictions do not include a blanket exclusion unless it is for good evidence-based reasons that you can support.
- Try to obtain or provide written information that may be given to patients explaining the reasons behind the decision.
- Ensure equitable access to any reduced service. This was predominantly a problem in relation to GP fundholders but will persist with primary care trusts and for as long as different authorities make different rationing decisions.
- Try to limit rationing to procedures not groups of people, that is, avoid hard boundaries, which can always be argued as illogical, but allow space for evidence-based medicine to have a role if its findings are explicit. For example, the denial of certain vascular surgical interventions to smokers, not because these smokers are smokers, but because the procedures will not work if they continue to smoke.
- Argue for services based on respect for humanity, not just simple life expectancy, even though this brings you back into the difficult area of "gender reassignment", infertility treatment, and mastopexy.
- Carry the clinicians with you.
- Always be prepared to revisit the decision.

6.4 IT/computers

The NHS is not a supermarket and it is not an airline. When it comes to IT (information technology) this is unfortunate. IT ought to be central to the smooth running of the NHS where 20–30% of employees' time is spent processing information, that is, where at any one time 250 000 people are handling data. Supermarkets and airlines, though less important to society than the NHS, are threaded through with sophisticated computer systems without which they would function less effectively or not at all. The NHS should be in their league but by any measure you care to take it is not only not winning it is not even playing. The NHS spends less than 0.5% of turnover on IT each year, which is substantially less than the 2% of turnover that commercial organisations expect to spend. The Audit Commission looked at the use of IT in NHS hospitals and found to no one's surprise that it was unsatisfactory. It did, however, produce a useful analysis of the failure, pointing out among other problems the lack of clinical leadership.[15]

As doctors and particularly as doctor-managers you will daily be frustrated by the incompatibility and inadequacies of the computer systems you will have to rely on; their age, their lack of sophistication, their slow unsympathetic formats. Rather than just complain and walk away you ought to do your bit to try and make it better, because it is doctors and doctors in management who I would submit are partly to blame for the present unhappy situation.

The underlying problem

Outsiders say that the computer problem in the NHS is fourfold. It is inadequately capitalised, there is a lack of clarity about what is needed, a lack of central authority to guide development, and a lack of good staff to implement it. Something that is politely summarised as "an immature business environment".

The arguments about the central control of computing development may in fairness be played either way, for or against. It is easy to construe as a stupendous failure the fact that the NHS did not see years ago the need to develop software to match the basic needs that are common to all hospitals; software that would allow one hospital and organisation to talk to another by use of the same data sets, the same security arrangements, etc. What one may assume to have been simply financial or planning cowardice could equally, however, be viewed historically as prudence, for what sallies into central planning there have been tended to have unhappy outcomes if the blind and malodorous alley of the Read code debacle is anything to go by. Despite this, the NHS is now set on a new and radical IT strategy to help deliver *The NHS Plan*. At its centre is a plan for "ruthless standardisation", with national standards for data sets and for system specifications. Billions of pounds are promised to make it all happen in partnership with software and hardware manufacturer consortia. There are problems with the devolved habits of IT development currently favoured as we shall see in a moment but centralised specification development and purchasing runs the risk of replicating on a truly magnificent scale all the disasters that can characterise IT developments.

IT in your hospital

Most hospitals have an IT department; either a man and his techno-dog or a bigger one with grander but more opaque titles such as "deputy systems engineer" ("No it's not my job to fix your PC") and "corporate network planner" ("No you can't connect your PC to the internet"). What many lack is a clear purpose.

The clear IT purpose (or lack of)

If your hospital's IT strategy is clear and workable and works, well done! (can I have a second opinion, please doctor?), but *don't* skip to the next chapter, things can still go wrong. If your hospital's IT strategy is, heaven forbid, less than clear, then as like or not you will find it has been jointly drafted by a senior computer nerd, the director of finance, and a doctor brought in "because he/she knows about computers" (that is, has one at home). What should perhaps have happened is something like this.

Stage One   Strategy should be set based purely on management and clinical criteria. No computer input is needed at this stage and I would beg to suggest that there is an advantage at this stage of excluding anybody with an interest in or knowledge of computers. Only when the needs have been defined as a brief prioritised list should the computer people be set loose on it.

Stage Two   Now it gets more difficult because having defined the outline requirements of what you want you will need, in consultation with the computer people, to decide for each problem:

- whether it *can* be computerised
- whether it *needs* to be computerised
- whether it needs to link with other systems
- where in the sequence of developments it will be placed.

There are separate strands here which need to be interwoven as the process evolves. A computer person will need to ensure that a system can be achieved within the defined cost and is technically feasible and a clinician/manager/nurse, etc will need to define the exact user specification. In this last context in my experience it has been very difficult to recruit doctors to spend the considerable time and energy on system development that is needed at the specification stage, and if you do recruit someone it is often difficult to get them to fix on what is practical and achievable. The detailed "Statement of Need" produced for a new test ordering and reporting system for our trust ran to 87 pages. That sort of effort requires real time and commitment from clinicians.

Most hospital trusts need computing for 10 core activities.

1. Payroll.
2. Personnel.
3. Patients' master index.
4. Finance.
5. Scheduling of theatres, clinics, radiographs, etc.
6. Ordering tests and seeing the results.
7. Waiting list management.
8. Bed management.
9. Core information (clinical protocols, drug data, etc).
10. Communication.

These are all products that require an endpoint. You will find that many of your colleagues are keen to record all sorts of audit and activity data on computer and may need to be reminded that high-volume ephemeral data in general costs more to enter than is justified and is rarely retrieved.

There is an enormous amount of data in any healthcare system. The Audit Commission estimates that about a quarter of doctors' and nurses' time is spent collecting and using data.[16] What part of this would be better managed with the use of computer systems is unknown. Enthusiasts will say that it is self evident that computers must be used for all these tasks but Lock, in a review of the published literature,[17] found only scanty objective evidence to support that view. He concluded that certain benefits are, however, likely to accrue from the use of computers and cited:

- easier access to the medical history and the results of tests
- easier and quicker generation of letters and discharge summaries
- support for protocols and guidelines
- support for shared care between professionals.

Some current and expensive developments such as PACS (picture archiving and communication system) which seem to be concerned with imaging systems are really just another IT project needing all the planning, wide consultation, and adequate initial investment that other IT systems demand.

The role of the clinician-manager

Clinicians involved in planning systems need to use their clinical knowledge and experience to judge what information *needs* to be processed and to bear in mind that ideally data should be recorded in "real time" (when it happens) and the recording should be a normal part of clinical/managerial care. In the NHS, which has traditionally been labour intensive, we have a fixation on manually entered data: bar codes rarely get a look in. I am not saying all patients should have bar codes tattooed on their bottoms, but supermarkets handle huge volumes of data infinitely better than we do and the bar code is inseparable from that. We are told as usual that the capital cost prohibits progress.

Clinicians in management need to ensure that things go well when planning computer systems. I would submit that medical managers have a responsibility to be very hard-nosed—both with the IT department and more particularly with their colleagues when it comes to planning systems. Here are some questions that you might ask.

- Do we really need this system?
- Will it really save money? (This is not an absolute requirement but it helps to obtain the funding.)

You should be aware of the "boys with toys" phenomenon in computer systems. Clinicians are just as prone to this disease as non-clinicians, possibly more so. The "boys with toys" phenomenon obtains where individuals or a group decide they need a computer system because it seems interesting, exciting, up to date, or fashionable. Their enthusiasm may outrun managerial pragmatism. Infants always "need" the things they want. When trying to understand whether a need is genuine one may be frustrated by an unholy alliance between doctors who want the new toy, computer people inside who want a fashionable project, and suppliers outside who want the contract signed and who will promise the earth to get it. Remember what happened to Dr Faust and be very hard-nosed! You the manager are more dependent on computer outputs than other clinicians. You can only make effective decisions if you have accurate aggregated clinical data, so you need to ensure that systems are robust.

Here are some more hard-nosed questions to ask.

- Given the limited availability of finance do you want this system in preference to some other expenditure which is not computer related?
- Do the systems which you already have and which are central to your business actually work properly or would the money be better spent on improving them?
- Does the system you are proposing require planned replacement? If so how will you fund it?
- Will you be able to afford the support costs?
- Do you need staff specifically to run the system?

Sad to say, my experience is that however hard you try your organisation will buy at least one system that it cannot afford, does not need, and that does not work. You *will* be a victim.

You will be a victim

Most clinicians do not understand computer technology in any real way nor appreciate the speed of its change, nor have an in-depth understanding of what is achievable, so it is easy to take us for a ride. At the very least during that ride which may, of course, be exciting we should ask our helmeted, wild-eyed, Mr Toad who is driving about the following.

- *Software documentation*: will it be unavailable or available but incomprehensible as usual?
- *Support*: will it be adequate? Whizz kids whizz off elsewhere, software firms go bust or get taken over.
- *May we assume that the system you are implementing will always work more slowly than you want and security will be non-existent*: because Nurse Blogg's access code has been written in indelible ink beside the computer screen so that all the agency nurses can use it?
- *When the system needs to be expanded because the original specification was poorly written*: will there be enough digits in the codes, enough free hand space in the forms, and generally enough leeway in the software and the hardware?
- *Have you clearly identified the suppliers' liabilities if the system does not work as they claim*: have the suppliers tried contractually to limit their liabilities and have we taken steps to protect ourselves against that?

When eventually Mr Toad gets you to his destination and you emerge shaken and poorer but with a spanking new computer system make sure you have arranged to have an objective review in six months' or a year's time, and if it really is not good enough, appropriate enough, flexible enough, and is costing you more and more in support and modification have the perspicacity to junk it there and then.

I must apologise to the reader for this section having been couched in such negative terms, but as most of what you will read elsewhere about computers and computing in the NHS tends to skirt around the snags, no apology is really needed. One hopes new developments will be proportionately of more value for patients' care, for example telemedicine, the medical use of the internet, and features of the NHS network itself such as the National Electronic Library for Health (http://www.nelh.nhs.uk). There is good evidence that competent computer systems can make hospital health care more efficient and even cheaper.[18] There are lots of genuinely useful and exciting developments in computing within the NHS and the single message I would want to finish with is that doctors and doctor-managers have a critical role in ensuring that these developments are appropriate and workable, so do not be put off by what I have said above, just be wary.

6.5 Risk and risk management

We live in an age of fear; not real fear of death and starvation, penury and war but a corrosive anxiety that in any situation the worst will happen, that nothing is safe and no one and no thing or principle is to be trusted.[19] The environment that this insecurity spawns generates numberless attempts to regulate and check what has happened or what might happen and convoluted attempts to minimise any risk that an individual or organisation might fall prey to. The United States spends about $200 billion a year towards regulating health and safety and environmental risk. You could say this habit is simply wise caution or you could see it as a loss of trust and self confidence. Whatever your interpretation, it is for now a fact of life that one must manage risk actively and centrally. Between 1967 and 1972, "risk" was cited 1300 times in medical journals; between 1987 and 1992 "risk" was cited 110 000 times; between 1997 and 2002 this had jumped to a whopping 245 227 citations on PubMed. There are now journals, specialist lawyers, management advisers, and conference organisers all living off the phenomenon of "risk". As a doctor the major risks that will concern you are the risks to patients flowing from inept clinical care. A person in hospital faces a one in 200 risk of significant error compared with a one in 2 000 000 risk on an aeroplane.[20] There are also "Health and Safety" issues relating to the general hospital environment, the handling of toxic chemicals, waste disposal, fire escapes, etc, etc, etc. Hospitals were once under "Crown Immunity" which allowed them to take a cavalier approach to health and safety issues, but that immunity has gone; health and safety inspectors now visit hospitals, although since 1988 there were only a smattering of successful prosecutions for breaches of hygiene and for unsafe equipment. This small number probably simply reflected a softly softly approach by the Health and Safety Inspectorate. The pace is hotting up and in 1997 the Chief Executive of the Swindon and Marlborough Trust resigned after the trust was found guilty of a breach of health and safety regulations. That was a salutary lesson about hospitals' relationships with the National Audit Office as that trust was one of those voluntarily participating in a study of accidents in hospital by the National Audit Office. District auditors looked at accidents in 30 NHS acute trusts during May and June 1995.[21] They discovered that more than half the trusts did not have incident recording systems, but even so they felt able to calculate that there were about half a million accidents each year in acute hospital trusts in England and Wales. Three-quarters of the accidents involved patients and visitors, and 80% were due to slips, trips, and falls. Among the staff most of the recorded accidents were needlestick injuries (of which of course only a minute fraction are reported). Nurses take 360 000 days' sick leave per year for reasons of occupational health or injury. Only half of trusts comply with more than 70% of legislation on health and safety. Most of this is not your business as a clinical manager but the need to reduce *clinical* risk most emphatically is.

All hospitals need a *programme of risk management*. This does not mean importing expensive risk management consultants to tell you what you know or can find out for yourself but cannot afford to put right. Fundamentally, it means a drive to change the culture away from passive risk acceptance to active risk prevention.

"Risk management" sounds commercial even slightly disreputable, as if you cared about the risk to the organisation rather than the victim. Doctors are almost unwittingly involved in a continuous process of risk management all the time though on a small scale. Do I need to get a haemoglobin? Do all patients aged over 50 need a preoperative chest radiograph? Can I discount the possibility that this patient will have a side effect from the drug I am about to prescribe? What are the risks of not admitting this patient now but waiting until tomorrow? Risk management is simply that activity generalised onto the whole organisation's business. The phrase "risk management" is a good one because it accepts that risks cannot be obviated and that the organisation must admit the ever-present sword of Damocles but try to arrange its business to minimise the risk of it falling and minimise the damage when it does.

A considered review of most hospitals' risk environment would probably show that the string holding Damocles' sword has been sawn nine-tenths through and the bulk of the hospital staff and patients marshalled into a huddle directly beneath it. Hospitals are dangerous places, they are full of malevolent bacteria, surgeons, unrestrained technology, radiation, partly trained agency nurses, junior doctors half asleep, and equipment that is years beyond its date for replacement. Yet we affect not to notice. The real risk is that risk management is seen merely as another chore which will cost us money, upset people, and take up valuable time that could be better spent doing something else. The slightly pernickety, nannyish attitude of the bureaucrats who administer "health and safety" issues and their frequent inability to understand the hierarchy of risks in a hospital makes this the agenda item greeted with a groan.

Your organisation may have faced up to these issues, but if not a way forward might include the following.

1. Change the mind set of employees so that they see risks and faults not as the responsibility of reprehensible individuals but as an institutional issue requiring institutional solutions. Also change the attitude to error so as to see adverse events as valuable indicators of how the organisation functions at its core as well as at its tatty edges.

2. Establish a risk management committee. Yes I know it is another committee and we don't want extra committees but this is an exception. It should have on it at least the chief executive, the director of nursing and the medical director and should report either to the board or the executive. It may be appropriate to establish as a subcommittee a group of clinicians looking specifically at issues of *clinical* risk.

3. Examine all the areas of the institution's business (with help from outside consultants if you must) and identify high-risk areas. Prioritise them for action.

4. Set an action plan and explicitly require clinicians and managers to attend to the identified problems within a specified timescale.

5. Raise the general awareness of risk in the organisation by involving as many staff as possible in the process of risk assessment and management and by publishing your findings, actions, and outcomes.

6. Have a formal procedure available whereby staff may notify risks that they encounter.

7. Ensure that the director of finance understands that risk to patients equates to financial risk to the organisation, and persuade him/her that money spent on risk management is likely to save him/her money spent on litigation later.

The National Patient Safety Agency

When the first edition of this book was published in 1999 the above arrangements would have been an adequate response to risk management. In 2000 the document *An Organisation with Memory* was published which proposed a national system for reporting errors and a year later the government, as part of its process of extending central monitoring, ordered the establishment of NPSA (the National Patient Safety Agency). This agency collects data electronically, focusing on a no-blame context, and tries to find common threads that may be synthesised into warnings that may help trusts avoid similar mistakes in future. At the time of writing the agency was in the throes of teething troubles concerning not only the complex business of capturing the right data efficiently and effectively but also the political discomforts that arose from the publication of pilot data. The plan is for a lot of its data to be freely available to the public in future; it will be largely anonymous but there are considerable worries that mischief-making "investigative journalists" will have good sport with the data which will involve some finger pointing that will be far removed from the no-blame ethos that is intended to encourage frank reporting. The project will need watching carefully. The website address is http://www.npsa.nhs.uk.

Whatever the outcome it will be prudent for clinical managers to ensure that their own in-house systems remain robust.

High-risk areas

Many breaches of health and safety regulations or accidents are trivial, this is acknowledged by NPSA, which categorises incidents as red, orange, yellow or green, depending on the severity of risk to patients. High-risk areas are already well recognised but correcting these may require money, sometimes a lot of money; and there is no separately identified funding for this even if the NPSA highlights it. Trust managers have the unenviable task of assessing the severity of risk and then balancing the need for expenditure to reduce low-level risks to staff, patients, and visitors against more predictable benefits from spending the money on high-grade risks or on direct patient care. We are not allowed publicly to admit the frustrations of being told by health and safety people that such and such a risk, which we perceive as trivial, *must* be dealt with immediately; yet there is no finance to cover the cost. To inform them in the execution of this balancing act all trusts need explicit "risk management" arrangements and an awareness of the magnitude of the different risks in human terms.

Common sense, clinical knowledge, a review of litigation claims and of complaints will identify some common threads that run through the highest areas of real risk in most hospitals and other health institutions (Figure 6.5). In so far as the clinical care of patients is concerned, high-risk areas are as follows.

- Obstetrics and orthopaedics. In these there is a crucial need for agreed and adhered to protocols and close supervision of junior doctors.[22]
- Locums and their induction, agency nurses.
- Inadequate note keeping and storage of records.
- Uncorrected faults in equipment.
- Inadequate hand over from doctor to doctor and nurse to nurse at shift change.
- Activities outside the normal area for the institution.
- Inappropriate delegation and working beyond personal competence levels.
- Drug mistakes.
- Failure to act on the results of pathology and imaging tests.

Not all of these risks are, of course, truly within your province as a medical manager, but there are some areas where doctors need to take the lead, particularly in specifying who can be safely allowed to do what, for example how to flatten the nasty bit of the learning curve in endoscopic surgery. Some areas of risk may require you the clinical manager, now or in the future, to take some difficult decisions which are difficult to implement and which may widen the gulf between you and your clinical colleagues. The issue of relating volumes of a procedure undertaken to the clinical outcomes that leads on to certification and to deciding who shall and shall not be allowed to undertake procedures within a hospital is the most contentious in this area.[23] The most visible aspect of this is surgeons who perform a wide range of operations some of them only infrequently. We know from published data that, for example, there is a substantial excess mortality from

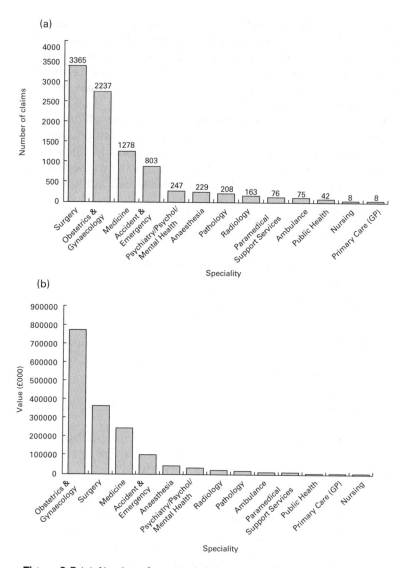

Figure 6.5 (a) *Number* of reported claims to the Clinical Negligence Scheme for trusts, subdivided by speciality. (From the NHS Litigation Authority annual report 2002, with permission.) (b) *Value* of reported claims to the Clinical Negligence Scheme for trusts, subdivided by speciality. (From the NHS Litigation Authority annual report 2002, with permission.)

undertaking only a small number of oesophagectomies or pancreatectomies a year. Most surgeons recognise this difficulty but it is difficult to stop and all sorts of specious arguments will be put to you, claiming for example that a particular individual's performance is better than average so they are safe or that they need to retain a breadth of experience so that they may be on-call. A more difficult area involves the undertaking of new or innovative procedures where being unwilling to take a risk will hamper progress.

We and lawyers tend to think of risk as being inherent in specifics, people, equipment or protocols, but we need to remember that there are features of the organisation itself which are recognised as increasing risk, in particular, rapid change, poor morale, inadequate communications, and a high workload.[24]

Indeed a "vulnerable system syndrome" has been identified that has three interacting and self-perpetuating elements:[25]

- blaming front-line individuals
- denying the existence of systemic promoting weaknesses
- the blinkered pursuit of productive and financial indicators.

The risks inherent in doctors' incompetence or illness are dealt with in Sections 4.7 to 4.9.

The costs of neglecting risk

Although only 0·5% of the NHS budget is spent on risk management, a successful claim against your trust can have potentially dramatic implications for its finances. It is not uncommon for obstetric claims to exceed £1 million. Of this the fraction representing 0·5% of the trust's annual revenue must be paid by the trust, the remainder must be borrowed from the Treasury and repaid with interest within 10 years. The NHS LA (NHS Litigation Authority) will negotiate structured settlements in these cases. NHS trusts are forbidden from taking out commercial insurance to protect themselves against these kind of risks but there exists the Clinical Negligence Scheme for Trusts (CNST) which is a cooperative system within the health service that helps to spread the risks.

Not everyone has joined this and it quite properly has some stringent entrance requirements requiring risk management procedures to be in place.

The future

Risk and error are not phenomena about to be "solved". The Harvard Medical Practice Study found 3·7% of admissions involved an adverse event, and in 1% of admissions care was judged to be negligent and to have contributed to permanent disability or the death of the patient.[26] That is probably a very low figure, an Australian study found that 16·6% of admissions resulted in an adverse event.[27] Another study proposed that there are 100 000 deaths per year in the USA from adverse drug reactions, a suspiciously round figure![28] Currently, only a tiny proportion of these are documented or acted upon. Even so it is claimed that it would cost as much as £4 billion to settle the UK's outstanding negligence cases.

Managing "adverse incidents"

This is an important and very practical issue for clinical directors, as being aware of these incidents, investigating them, and learning from them it is part of their clinical governance responsibilities. Firstly, they need to have an effective reporting system in place that all the staff feel confident to use because it is easy and does not lead to an exercise in blaming and punishing. Much of what is reported will be trivial and may be investigated by a junior manager and regularly reported to directorate meetings. More important events, such as those where a patient's death or serious injury occurs, must be addressed by clinical directors personally. The fact that there may be litigation or an inquest in the offing does not absolve them of the responsibility to act, though they will normally do so in concert with the risk management or complaints departments of the trust and will have been in touch with the medical director and/or director of nursing. For serious incidents there should be an inquiry. This should be formal, prompt, and led by an independent inquirer, usually a senior nurse and/or clinician who was not involved in the incident. They should be given formal terms of reference, should interview all involved parties, should ensure that the employees involved have made written statements about what happened, and lastly, must inspect all relevant notes. A formal report should be produced and inquirers should be prepared to discuss this in a constructive way with the staff involved and with the patient or their relatives. Importantly, if the inquiry finds no fault this should be stated, however difficult relatives or patients may be about that. They should not be cowed by claims of "whitewash" as the carefully garnered facts should protect them. What is interesting about all this is that, despite much international effort at reducing risk by reporting adverse incidents and learning from them, there is not yet any hard evidence to show that this strategy actually reduces those adverse events or is cost effective.

6.6 Education versus service

You would perhaps not expect to find a section on education in a book about clinicians and management. Most such books ignore it, yet experience as a medical manager shows that the impact of education on service and vice versa is an everyday and difficult problem. Indeed, clinicians in management may be on either side in the service versus education tussles, or even both, although rarely synchronously. For me the reality of the potential clashes was evident from the day when I became clinical director of surgery and was politely asked by my colleagues to give up the post of surgical tutor as the two posts were thought to have incompatible agendas.

Education versus service problems come up in two distinct areas.

1. The education of trainees.
2. Undergraduate training.

The most difficult of these is the first.

Service commitments of trainees

Trainee doctors train predominantly on the job and for generations service as apprenticeship was the norm, and in most instances was the best. Many clinicians, possibly most clinicians, still believe this model to be the best and there is research evidence to support that view. Nevertheless, the apprenticeship model which has lasted us well for many centuries is now under relentless pressure from reduced hours of work, from a faster turnover of patients, from a more "efficient" service which does not allow sufficient time for consultant and trainee to be together, and lastly, in many instances, from the trend to a "consultant-based" as distinct from a "consultant-led" service. It sometimes seems there is also a confounding problem in that educationalists may seem not to perceive any virtue at all in the apprenticeship system. We have then, on the one hand, a host of clinicians and indeed many trainees, especially surgical ones, who believe that simply getting on with the job and being supervised for a proportion of the time is the way to learn. Set against this, on the other hand, are educationalists who believe that all trainees should be surplus to service requirements, that training should be predominantly formal and structured, and that a good deal of it should be accrued away from the bedside. One has to be careful not to paint a picture of a battlefield that does not really exist, but these polarities are real so let us just say that the polarities lead to competing priorities for medical managers who are, once again, pigs in the middle and need to address the conflicts.

The champions of educational priorities are the SACs (Specialist Advisory Committees), postgraduate deans, universities, royal and other colleges, and the various visiting teams that they all spawn. The rules of best educational practice to which these teams work are an amalgam of educational theory, educational fashion, government directives, and financial rules concerning holding trainees' salaries. All of these are complicated and require special knowledge. These byways of the regulations associated with trainees are often bizarre, consisting of little known tracks between the NHS, universities, colleges, and medical schools. Special knowledge of this terrain breeds its own maquisards—small groups of activists—determined to stand up for education against the crushing forces of finance-driven service provision. They operate in small bands as visiting recognition teams. Pitched battles are rare, victories small but progressive. Behind many of them is the shadowy but inspirational figure of Le Patron, the regional postgraduate dean. He/she is important because he/she controls the weaponry, the money that pays for these trainees, and in part the recognition processes that allow hospitals to employ them. What are managers to do? The in-house finance people want efficiency savings and the purchasers want higher quality for lower cost and a consultant-based service. The colleges want more experience for trainees but the hours regulations have them working less. The university house officer inspection team wants the world to revolve around the house officer and newly empowered nurses want to take over the house officer's work. The whole jumble of competing requirements revolves on an endless merry-go-round. Every once in a while one of the teams comes to visit; you smile and wave and another comes by and you smile and wave until they have gone, because, in most instances, unfortunately you simply cannot square the circle. What each group wants is not compatible with what the other wants, so you smile and wave as they go by knowing that it will be at least a year before they are back and that most of their threats of withdrawal of recognition, etc simply are not implementable because everyone else has the same problem. This is a sadly cynical attitude to take but it has for a long time been an unhappy state of affairs although it is slowly improving. The regional postgraduate deaneries are trying to ensure that incompatible demands are not made by different visiting teams, but unfortunately purchasers of health care (and that includes the Department of Health at origin) do not have mechanisms in place to ensure that adequate and funded time is set apart for both trainees and consultants to engage in formal educational processes. What they have done by contrast is insist that education occurs during the working week. The European Working Hours Directive will in time reduce the week to 48 hours, which will add yet another dimension of difficulty to the problem (*see* Section 6.7).

The solutions to all this will, in the predictable future, have to remain compromises. The point at which service yields to education and vice versa will no doubt move in a pendulum fashion. In the meantime the best medical managers can do about it is not to see it as a battle, to remain on good terms with the educational teams, and when involved in business planning they will need to do their best to write in the time and costs of education and keep education on the agenda, not only with the managerial side of the organisation but also with the clinicians.

That is very bland and will probably be insufficient in some areas where there will indeed be a battle between service and education which may resolve itself in two ways. The one most often threatened is that clinicians who do not teach and organisations who do not educate will lose their right to have trainees. Indeed it is possible that whole hospitals may in future be manned by consultants and "non-career grade" staff. For the educationalists there is of course also a risk of brinkmanship in that hospitals may say, as mine once had to about house surgeons in the "New Deal", that the difficulties produced by the requirement to train and meet the hours requirements were so great that it was no longer in the organisation's interests to continue to offer that training. Many junior doctor tasks are now satisfactorily undertaken by nurses, and if their role is looked at completely cold-bloodedly, without any sympathy to the overall educational needs of the service, then they might indeed be considered expendable. The bluff worked.

At the other end of training there are anxieties for medical managers that graduates from the new SpR training process are not sufficiently trained to take on consultant posts. This is far from a theoretical worry and posts are already remaining unfilled, not through lack of applicants but through lack of properly trained applicants. Many of the trainees realise that this is a risk but are caught by the guillotine of European legislation which does not enable training to continue beyond what it decrees appropriate. One is always wary of identifying more resources as the solution to problems, but most people conclude that the only solution to the current educational difficulties is to have sufficient extra staff available at consultant level to enable more formal educational time with trainees. There will in addition need to be structured education for trainers. Doctors are not professional teachers and they need to be taught to teach and to assess. Until that happy day medical managers will have to continue to orchestrate the compromises.

Undergraduate teaching

Medical managers cannot become distanced from issues of undergraduate teaching and simply assume that it is the medical school's job. Many hospitals, not just teaching hospitals, receive money from a mechanism known as SIFT (Service Increment for Teaching) that is destined to meet the extra NHS costs associated with teaching medical and dental undergraduates. This is added in most cases to budgets which medical managers may feel are clinical budgets. In the past it was simply an item in the allocation, but since 1999 allocation of this money depends on a bottom up assessment of true costs of providing extra resources for undergraduate teaching.

If they are involved in that unpicking, medical managers will need to cost items such as clinicians' undergraduate teaching sessions, the reduced number of patients seen in a teaching outpatients clinic, the provision of facilities for students to be taught in, the extra days of stay sometimes required so that patients can be taught on, etc. This is another of the unhelpful time-consuming exercises in unpicking costs, a process which everyone resents as they see no likely benefit in it.

6.7 Shifts and reduced working hours

On 1 August 2004 junior doctors in the National Health Service and other healthcare systems throughout Europe will no longer be excluded from the provisions of the European Working Time Directive ... This will demand even more profound changes for the NHS than seen so far in the long march for better working conditions for junior hospital doctors ... Unlike the new deal, the European Working Time Directive is not a gentleman's agreement. It is health and safety law, and we have less than 1000 days to comply.

(Pickersgill T. Editorial. *BMJ* 2001;**323**:1266.)

The gloating editorial by Pickersgill, the chairperson of the BMA's Junior Doctors Committee, convinces me that the *BMJ* is now the magazine for the coffee table of the politically active lily-livered doctors who populate the NHS. The smile will be wiped off Pickersgill's face if ever he is unfortunate enough to need an operation.

(Scott-Coombes D. Letter. *BMJ* 2002;**324**:736.)

One of the most intractable problems facing clinical directors is the impact of the "New Deal" arrangements for reducing trainees hours and of implementing the EWTD (European Working Time Directive)[29], a situation made more difficult by the seeming inability of the Department of Health to understand or to plan or budget effectively for the consequent disruption of clinical care and education. Indeed, the best it could offer in a guidance document issued in January 2003 was to suggest "creative redesign" of working patterns. Let us look at the hard facts first: the EWTD requires that all countries must have a 58 hour week in place by August 2004, 56 hours from 2007, and 48 hours from 2009 (but with a possible extension of the 56 hour week to 2012) but adds that junior doctors must have a minimum 11 hours' continuous rest after 13 hours on duty and 24 hours' continuous off duty for every seven days (or 48 for every fortnight). The European Court of Human Rights SIMAP ruling, the so called "Spanish clause", indicates that from August 2004 all hours spent at your place of work count as work even if you are resting, sleeping or studying. Time spent out of the hospital on-call at home only counts when services are actually being provided. At present increasingly stringent financial penalties are being applied in the form of extra payments from trusts' budgets if junior doctors work long hours. As a manager you have a number of options in dealing with this several of which you will need to deploy concurrently.

- You can change the shift pattern of the trainees to a partial shift or even to a full shift.
- You can arrange the work so that when clinicians are in the hospital they are always working, that is, no rest periods are rostered.
- You can employ extra clinical staff either in mainstream grades or in grades which do not suffer the same problems of surveillance and approval, such as staff grade doctors, trust doctors or clinical fellows.
- You can change the pattern of clinical work of consultants so that they spend more time in front-line activities, even on-call out of hours.
- You can downgrade the level of cover so that, for example, SpRs cover from home or SHOs and even SpRs cross-cover other specialities.
- You can arrange for nurses to cover some of the out of hours on-call work.
- You can merge departments between hospitals so that specialist and emergency teams become larger.

Whilst these are rational and appealing for managers, clinicians are aware of the risks which flow from a mechanical attitude to hours. In particular, losses of continuity of care, a tendency to postpone decisions for the next shift, delays in decision making for inpatients, a "clocking-off" mentality in the next generation of doctors and a worsened quality of life even though overall hours are shorter.[30] Studies are already showing the dire effects on training which even more formalised educational habits will have difficulty in offsetting. Crucially, the time spent at the bedside with a more senior person is reduced, longitudinal perception of patients' illnesses is rarely achieved, feedback to trainees about the appropriateness or effects of their management of emergency patients is impaired, and lastly, the opportunities for learning practical skills are reduced. This last is particularly critical for surgical trainees whose log books increasingly show inadequate exposure to opportunities for learning technical skills and who, as a consequence, are having to seek ways of extending their training after they have allegedly become fully accredited. The irony in this is that a change in working practice, which in part sprang from a desire to avoid harm to patients that might be caused by the lapses of tired doctors, may end up achieving the exact opposite effect quite apart from in some ways producing a poorer overall quality of life in its broadest sense, for doctors in training.

Full shift working

Like it or not this will invariably become the only workable solution for many trainees in the acute specialities. As a way of working it is increasingly common in society and has, of course, been normal for nurses for many years. As a result there is a lot of information available as to what steps managers can take to make such patterns more acceptable to staff. A literature review by Wilson[31] included the following recommendations.

- Use forward rotations of shift in a clockwise direction, that is, follow a sequence of morning shifts with afternoon ones and then nights. Avoid afternoon/evening shifts followed by morning shifts.
- Do not start daytime shifts before 8 am.

- Night shifts should be shorter than day shifts.
- There should always be at least two days off after a period of night shifts if accumulative fatigue is to be avoided.
- Staff must be involved in the planning of shifts and allowed choice or to negotiate "swaps" to minimise social disruption.
- Shift patterns should be as regular as possible.

To these recommendations one might add the following.

- Rosters should be defined well in advance and notified to staff well before they take up a post.
- Overlap between shifts of at least an hour must be allowed to ensure adequate handover.
- Define in writing how study leave and holidays are to be dealt with and what contingency arrangements will apply when staff are off sick.
- Allow staff to devise a better, though of course "legal" and workable, plan from yours if they wish.
- Remember that different specialities have different attitudes to the various solutions to this conundrum[32] (Figure 6.6).

There is even a website with software to help you plan, change, and disseminate rotas (http://www.rotadoc.com).

6.8 Audit, evidence-based medicine, and managed care

Thou wilt also learn one piece of Humility, viz. not to trust too much on thy own judgement.

(Richard Wiseman, Severall Chirurgicall Treatises, 1676.)

I have no failure to record, if we exclude the recurrences which I have reported and which could not be ascribed to my method.

(William Halstead on his method of Hernia repair.
Ann Surg 1893;**19**:542–56.)

Doctors' freedom to choose what they believe to be appropriate management for their patients is increasingly

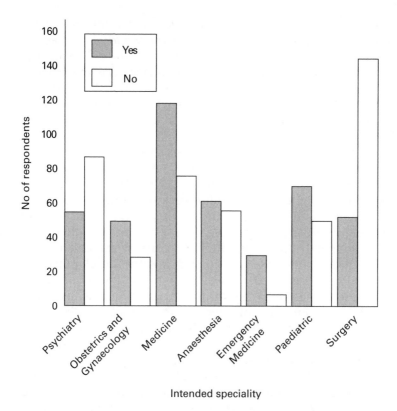

Figure 6.6 SHOs' and SpRs' preferences for working 13 hour shifts in a 56 hour week, by speciality. Essentially, this is a referendum on the acceptability of a full shift system of working—rejected by surgeons as incompatible with adequate training.[32] (From Aitken and Paice.)

being modified. There are several drivers to change in this area; they have evolved over the last 10 years to the point where no clinician can claim ignorance and no one is uninvolved. They are sometimes represented as a progressive erosion of clinicians' priest-like individual power and may thus be a source of conflict between doctors and managers. It is important for medical managers to understand the possible benefits and disbenefits of what is being done, as they are often the fulcrum about which the anxieties of clinicians and the aspirations of non-clinical managers rotate.

One might simplify this rolling revolution as follows. Firstly, there is a point of departure which is the *historical omnipotence of the clinician*. Even though as early as the time of Hippocrates the variability of practice between clinicians was understood, as was the inappropriateness of some of what they did, and even though the development of the scientific method allowed some analysis of this, the principle of "the doctor knows best" generally held sway. Only in the second half of the last century was the notion of individual doctors as the prime movers in patients' care seriously challenged. The challenge came from two directions: firstly, an appreciation that poor clinical outcomes might reflect faulty investigation, diagnosis or treatment; and secondly, that some investigations and treatments are more expensive than others and are often used inappropriately, that is, there are both quality and cost aspects.

In the UK, the response to this was the development of clinical audit as a peer review activity; either as a regular in-house exercise for the clinical team or nationally as in the Confidential Enquiry into Perioperative Deaths (CEPOD). In the USA, overutilisation was the predominant theme and indeed was the predominant problem. The trend there was towards professional review with mandatory second opinion or professional reviewers to check that the investigations, treatment, and lengths of stay remained within predefined limits. This was, and is, essentially a cost containment exercise which merely substitutes the views of one doctor or group of doctors for that of another. The second opinion was presumed to be more educated or biddable about the cost:benefit ratio than the first opinion. What has gradually emerged, curiously late in history, is that doctors as a group may know better than others how to treat disease, but individual doctors often do not know or apply the best management of disease—not through laziness or incompetence but simply through an inability to store, process and use the huge amounts of information that relate to disease and its management. Lawrence Weed has written about this,[33] and explicitly identifies the problem as "a misplaced faith in the unaided human mind" and that "until now we have believed that the best way to transmit knowledge from its source to its use in patient care is to first load the knowledge into human minds (the long and expensive education of professionals) and then expect those minds at great expense to apply the knowledge to those who need it. However there are enormous 'voltage drops' along this transmission line for medical knowledge" and that therefore "good medical practice requires tools to extend the human mind's limited capacity to recall and process large numbers of relevant variables" and that "these tools should be kept up to date and used routinely—not in heads which are expensive to load and faulty in the attention and processing of knowledge".

This would seem to be self evident, yet we continue to rely heavily on a high-quality, up-front education, and accreditation processes. Even with continuing postgraduate medical education the level of knowledge of most individuals is probably inadequate for all but the highest level of hyperspeciality. Doctors in general are also handicapped by their difficulty in convincing themselves that they would accept external constraints on the untrammelled power of their own memories/intuitions/skills to make crucial judgments about management. Hence the need for an audit process.

Audit

There is everything to be said in favour of the *principles* of clinical audit. All it asks is that clinicians critically review the results of their work on a regular basis, compare those results with those of others, and if there are lessons to be drawn, change their practice. This describes the classic feedback loop of audit which turns into a repeating cycle or spiral to improve quality (Figure 6.7). These corrective feedback loops were thought to be the solution to the defects in our knowledge, but the audit process in day-to-day use has proved to be a blunt and cumbersome tool. Audit, even aided by computers, clerks, and audit officers, is only able to focus on a few problems at a time and experience shows that the feedback loop from measurement to changed practice to remeasurement is only rarely completed and, even when it is, it works very slowly. A National Audit Office report published in 1995[34] reviewed nearly 7000 audit projects and looked in detail at 1441 undertaken at eight trusts. It found lots of audit activity underway (as there should have been given the £61 million cost)—most had involved confirmation of the benefits of care, changes in the process of care or the production of guidelines. Sadly, only one in six projects had gone around the whole audit

Figure 6.7 The audit cycle.

cycle and was being repeated. Evidence of specific benefit to patients was skimpy. By 2001 things were not much better[35] and there was still not much evidence of significant benefit to patients.[36]

It is customary to blame the failures of audit on the resistance of clinicians and their supposed unwillingness to have their shortcomings laid bare among their peers[37] or else to blame doctors for subverting the process so as to maintain their dominance in the system[38] or perhaps more honestly to admit that the methodology never matched the rhetoric.[39] What has interfered with the ability of audit to engage either our hearts or our minds is a frustration with the cumbersomeness of the audit process itself, the obviousness of the conclusions, and the powerlessness of the average clinician to change many of the causative defects in process. Audit has simply not had significantly more effect on day-to-day clinical practice than the normal evolution of professional knowledge would have done. Additionally, it has squandered stupendous quantities of medical time and sensitised a whole generation of trainee doctors against the process, largely one suspects because the system *demands* that we "do audit". Audit did not deliver the goods, so along came the armies of EBM (evidence-based medicine), whose cavalry has in most engagements quickly outflanked the dour and portly foot soldiers of the audit team.

The failures of audit

Audit as a core activity has been described as:

a vicious circle, a noose to strangle any chance of it ever being a practical every-day tool ... a whole service industry has mushroomed around this fatal flower, and with every new blossom it becomes more and more remote from real practice and from the people who are actually doing the work.[40]

That is overstated; nevertheless, a careful paper by Anthony Hopkins has analysed the reasons why audit has failed to win over the professionals.[41] He concluded that the problem is a conflict between clinical audit as a tool for education and professional development and its use for monitoring performance. He says in his summary:

it is my belief that the simple methods sufficient to improve care in a local and low key way have been confused with the much more rigorous methods required to monitor contract performance and to begin to compare the performance of different hospital teams. A great deal of money has been spent on employing audit assistants with insufficient knowledge of the complexities of clinical measurement and yet who try to impose this insufficiency of knowledge on the informal methods of directorate audit. No-one can criticise the NHS Executive for failing to provide financial resources to help first medical and then clinical audit, but this money was thrown at the problem without a sufficient research base in clinical audit, without sufficient attention to the social structures in hospitals and medical schools, and without sufficient recognition of the constructively critical faculties of health professionals.

That is, good principle, shame about the practice.

The ultimate irony for audit is that the benefits and cost effectiveness of audit have never themselves been properly audited; "we will never really know whether the national policy on clinical audit had a positive effect overall or whether the money could have been better spent. Audit will always be an act of faith."[42]

We should not leave audit on a negative note. Audit as an activity is growing up. The principle that guides it is sound, and slowly it is becoming better focused. One way of controlling it may be to commission specific audits from outside "suppliers" ("outsourcing" if you want to use management speak). There are several purely commercial organisations who will now do this for a fee but many professional groups have now established their own audits, to which their members contribute data, that can quickly show whose performance is below par though they may be less good at showing when we are doing the wrong thing. One thing that must be apparent even to those most irritated by the pedantic ways of in-hospital audit is that much of the change that is occurring around us is indeed in need of audit in a more general sense. Radical and expensive changes in clinical practice, such as the widespread adoption of laparoscopic surgery, has gone largely unaudited. Few of the predicted benefits of laparoscopic cholecystectomy seem to have accrued[43] and yet it is a procedure which in prospect seemed very likely to have both health and economic benefits. Even so only 11 of 1500 publications on it in English up to 1994 were randomised trials[44] and by then the technique was so entrenched that there was no prospect of that sort of study. As in so many areas there has been little evidence of the much needed clinical and managerial audit which should validate the implementation of new technology.

Confidentiality of audit records

Medical managers have not only a duty to ensure that audit is occurring effectively in their area but also must ensure that confidentiality is maintained for both patients or, "where appropriate", staff. Although it is claimed that clinical audit data is part of an educational process and its records are not available to lawyers seeking to use them, this is, in fact, not so in reality. There is no specific protection for these records and there is no specific law relating to the disclosure of clinical audit information in the UK. A test case will be required to settle any legal issues which might arise.[45]

Evidence-based medicine

Nothing, of course, is new and for all that its acolytes claim that EBM is a unique event in medical history, it is not. There have been plenty of empiricist, epistemic, and scientific doctors practising during the last 1000 years who have managed to improve the quality of medical care through careful assessment of the available evidence. Anyone who feels that the current debate about EBM is new might usefully read Rangachari's paper "Evidence based medicine: old French wine with a new Canadian label?",[46] in which he charts Pierre Louis' epistemic approach to the efficacy of blood letting in the management of disease and the positive and negative responses to his publications. All this was occurring in the first half of the nineteenth century. The clash then between the disciples of Louis' enthusiasm for the empirical approach versus the Gnostic clinicians' approach looking to the individual and human variability is exactly mirrored in papers of the 1990s. The philosophy underpinning EBM is simply the extension of a long historical thread that started when Newton and Descartes declared an overweening concern with observation, method, order, and pattern to the exclusion of individuality.

The introduction and discussion sections of any clinical scientific publication have always aimed at educating the clinician to make "the conscientious, explicit and judicious use of current best evidence in making decisions about the care of individual patients", which in fact, is the definition of EBM given by Sackett.[47] The definition by Sackett is a clinician's definition, but much the same as Appleby's definition of EBM as "the rigorous evaluation of the effectiveness of health care interventions, common dissemination of the results of the evaluation and use of the findings to influence clinical practice".[48] Appleby's definition is subtly different and a manager's definition, but it is all good worthy stuff which arguably has been around for as long as there have been scientists and managers. What is new, however, apart from a certain holier than thou gloss on the process, is the following.

1. The process of assessing the evidence has become more systematic and statistical and in the hands of statisticians rather than clinicians.

2. The results of the analysis are deliberately refined into clinical guidelines.
3. The process has been taken up (hijacked you might say) by public health doctors, managers, purchasers, and even the general public.
4. Changes in information technology have allowed easier dissemination of the conclusions, for example, the Cochrane database and the internet.
5. The process has also looked at structural issues, such as whether a higher flow of patients with a specific disease through a unit will produce better results.[49]

The central tenet of EBM is that a sophisticated analysis of the available data will yield a truth about the management of disease that can be the starting point for clinical guidelines which clinicians *ought* to use. The process even allows the guidelines to be annotated with an indication of the strength of the evidence that supports each recommendation. Levels of evidence quoted are:

- Ia   meta-analysis
- Ib   at least one controlled randomised trial
- II   at least one well-designed non-randomised trial
- III non-experimental descriptive studies, such as comparative or case studies
- IV   "respectable opinion".

It is a big leap from level I evidence, which is often scanty, to a workable guideline, so the views of professional groups, of patients, and of local users need to be integrated into any guidelines. This makes for a quasi-democratic product but not necessarily a clear one. Nevertheless, lots of guidelines are produced and in the process the scientific evidence on which we base our practice is sieved and graded and made available from sources such as the Cochrane database.

Crucially, guidelines must include local input, as people are suspicious of guidelines defined and imposed by people they do not know. By analogy Dr Muir Gray likes to tell the story of Mary Baker who invented the first instant cake mix but found it did not sell until the powdered egg ingredient was omitted and the person making the cake contributed by breaking into the mix their own, real raw egg.[50]

Box 6.1 Checklist for desirable attributes when assessing guidelines

- Validity
- Cost effectiveness
- Reproducibility
- Reliability
- Patient and user involvement
- Clinical applicability
- Clinical flexibility
- Clarity
- Meticulous documentation
- Scheduled review date linked to audit

Once guidelines are available they not only afford a core of reliable information to guide clinicians but they also help to improve communication with patients and other professionals who can all be working from the same data which is particularly important in the context of the discontinuous care now provided because of reduced working hours (Box 6.1). They improve risk management by identifying areas where training or supervision is needed. Guidelines, in theory, may improve the effective use of our resources. They can additionally identify research and audit needs. This all sounds optimistic but the guidelines have been shown genuinely to have these effects.[51]

The production of guidelines is, nevertheless, a laborious process and guidelines are not yet available for all eventualities, but we are getting there. A brave new era has dawned. The triumph of rationality and shared experience over ignorance and conservatism! Or is it? *Truth* as the French philosopher Michel Foucault observed is not something real and permanent but something "produced" by an elite as part of a "system of exclusion" of alternative options.

Problems with evidence-based medicine

There is much spoken and published criticism of EBM. Some just, some unjust based on a misunderstanding of what it is about. It is hardly surprising that there should be opposition; the term EBM itself implies that other medicine is not evidence based, which is clearly not true, although EBM afficionados love to repeat the completely untested axiom that 90% of what doctors do has no scientific basis. What is primarily at stake is the legitimacy of the evidence advanced to support a decision about a patient's management. The quality of evidence which underpins EBM is on the surface exceptionally good, deliberately so, and thus its legitimacy would seem to be secure, but there is a danger in placing too much importance on the results of published clinical trials and then generalising them to the whole population. There is evidence to show that such published trials are biased in favour of interventional procedures and those with positive results. Multiple publications of the same data will also bias a result. Negative results tend not to be published,[52] as are studies looking at qualitative issues such as the attitudes and perceptions of patients, because these are not easy to grind in the statistical mill.[53] A population study must be clearly defined and tends to exclude the aged and those with comorbidity. The quest in EBM has been for "internally valid" evidence, that is, scientifically pure, to the exclusion of "externally valid", that is, generally applicable evidence.[54] More worrying, perhaps, are nagging anxieties about the crown jewel of EBM, the meta-analysis.[55] In the past we were warned about the dangers of combining disparate studies if we wished to have a believable result and combining disparate studies is what meta-analysis does. One study analysed meta-analyses for the sort of biases mentioned above and found bias in 38% of meta-analyses published in four leading journals.[56] Unfortunately, there is no statistical way of resolving the problem of heterogeneity,[57] nevertheless a careful meta-analysis may indeed be the best means that we possess to assess the available data; its great danger is that its conclusions will be believed and that having "lumped" together the data we will forget to "split" it apart again when applying the conclusions to different patients.[58] The mechanics of the analysis are so opaque to the mere clinician or manager that what is concluded is likely to be taken as gospel even though it may quite simply be wrong. Le Lorier and his team in Montreal looked at instances where large randomised trials had addressed the same questions as previous meta-analyses. They found that in 35% of the instances studied the findings of the randomised study differed from those predicted by the meta-analysis.[59] Hence a need not only for obsessional care about the processes of meta-analysis itself but also for great scepticism and even greater care when promulgating guidelines.[60,61]

I am sorry to go on like this about EBM, there is really nothing wrong about it in principle but as a medical manager you need to understand its limitations because all too often you will be expected to sell protocol'd, EBM-based care to your colleague clinicians who will often have a more sophisticated view of EBM than the manager who wants you to whip the team into line; they may see it simply as one of many tools rather than something "holding top position in a delusional hierarchy of evidence".[62,63]

At the risk of boring you let us pursue this a little further.

Consensus and guidelines

The clinician unlike the basic scientist has to act even when knowledge is insufficient for a fully informed decision. A "consensus" view under these circumstances can be achieved in only three ways: by compromise, by selection of an expert panel whose views conform, or by use of language that obscures differences.

When there are genuine differences of opinion in a review panel, compromise is the only way in which apparent unanimity can be obtained. The objection to describing the result as a consensus is that the term carries an authority that "compromise guidelines" would not. Bias in selection of a review panel is unlikely to be intentional, but nevertheless carries an important risk. Distinction in medical science reflects prevailing values and prejudices; the minority questioning voice may well not be selected, although it may belong to tomorrow's majority.

(Editorial[60])

But we need guidelines

Whatever their shortcomings we need guidelines as one of the ways by which quality of care can be improved, if for no other reason than that doctors not only may not know what is current best treatment but may not know that they don't know.[64] More importantly the use of publicised best practice is the surest way for the public to be assured that they are being properly treated. There are a large number of groups working to produce best practice guidelines, some national and some local. The need for comprehensiveness and consensus leads to guidelines being sometimes vague (*might, may, could* featuring often) and the time taken for their completion and propagation can lead to them being out of date. For example, the Royal

College of Surgeons of England's first guidelines on hernia repair advocated the Shouldice technique, but was instantly rendered meaningless by the publication of the first large series showing the excellence of the Lichenstein mesh repair; information available to readers of the surgical journals but not available to those reading only the guidelines! But the most cogent criticism is that guidelines do not sit comfortably with the hurly burly of daily clinical practice where doctors have to address not diagnoses but clinical problems, for example not angina but chest pain, and the guidelines are written for angina. Additionally, the guidelines are global and not specific and may not be appropriate for the old patient with concurrent problems or the GP as distinct from the hospital doctor. Lastly, they can subvert the cultural importance of the *art* of medicine, which involves understanding the whole patient from a physical, psychological, and social perspective; treatment being based as much on experience and intuition as on a purely scientific approach. Thirty years ago Lord Platt wrote: "I am therefore somewhat concerned lest the extreme believer in the creed of scientific medicine should be bringing up a generation of doctors who can no longer trust their own observations or their judgement".[65] Many of us still share that anxiety:

> the presence of reliable evidence does not ensure that better decisions will be made. Claims that evidence based medicine offers an improved method of decision making are difficult to evaluate because current practice is so poorly defined. Medical decision making draws upon a broad spectrum of knowledge—including scientific evidence, personal experience, personal biases and values, economic and political considerations, and philosophical principles (such as concern for justice), it is not always clear how practitioners integrate these factors into a final decision, but it seems unlikely that medicine will ever be entirely free of value judgements.

> (Kerridge et al.[66])

Does this matter? Well yes it can. If EBM were simply an exercise by doctors and academics for winnowing the mass of information that has accumulated then it would probably be safe. But the use of EBM has gone far beyond that. We may argue the scientific rights and wrongs of EBM but it is the inappropriate use of EBM for managerial purposes that is worrying, and it is here that medical managers need to ensure

Figure 6.8 The position of EBM as merely one of the inputs into the clinical decision making process. (From Haynes *et al.*)

that sense prevails. Someone must not only judge the protocol itself but also decide when a departure from protocol was not simply ignorance, and someone must have the wit to see when protocols are strangling innovation or humanity (Figure 6.8).

Rules are for the obedience of fools and the guidance of the wise.

(Anon)

EBM and medical managers

In December 1993 an NHS Executive Letter (93/115) was issued covering "a developing initiative to integrate professional guidelines more effectively into the delivery of health care" and "to develop guidelines which will be useful in framing discussions between purchasers and providers on the development of service specifications and contract negotiations". EBM had moved from a clinical tool to a managerial one. That is not necessarily a bad thing, but clinicians in management now have a crucial role to ensure that non-clinicians wishing to use EBM guidelines understand their inadequacies and the potential dangers of their too rigid use. Dangers encapsulated, for example, in the notion that "clinical *effectiveness*" requires unstinting adherence to the guidelines, and that departure from them implies clinical *ineffectiveness*. EBM guidelines are, of course, valuable for suggesting an expected form of treatment with which to bring clinicians and units using outdated or less effective therapies up to date, but their unvarying use for every patient in a single unit carries hazards. Medical managers need to ensure that clinical practice does not become "tyrannized by evidence"[67] so that everything is judged only against the guidelines and not seen in context.

I am not suggesting that medical managers becomes "Horatio On The Bridge" holding back barbarian hoards of EBM-crazed managers, simply that they are clear in their own minds of the benefits and dangers of EBM. They may also need to police the production of guidelines locally. There is also the difficult issue of the legal position of guidelines and the anxiety that doctors have that departures from guidelines might weaken their position in any complaint or legal action against them. It is a complex area but the "Bolam test" will still apply and that doctors' actions in any specific context are thus likely to be judged by whether a responsible body of peers would have acted in a similar way. The existence of professionally agreed guidelines will, however, certainly make it more difficult to justify departures from them, and it is expected that they will in time erode the Bolam principle which has guided medicolegal decisions for so many years. The Bolitho case may be the first step down that road. The Law Lords in deciding this appeal opined that the court has to be satisfied that "the exponents of a body of opinion relied on could demonstrate that such opinion had a logical basis".[68]

The legal ramifications of writing or using guidelines are as you would expect complex but a good summary can be found in a paper by Tingle.[69]

Clinical managers also need to remember that too close a public adherence to guidelines can for many patients smack of medical authoritarianism and force them into the hands of alternative practitioners.

Lastly, medical managers need to consider how guidelines may be moved from paper to practice. The implementation of guidelines is the implementation of change and the obstructions to change are usually people and their attitudes, sometimes also resources. Attitudes to change are more often conditioned by beliefs than by evidence and changing peoples' beliefs is difficult.[70,71]

In summary: 10 action points

Internally

1. *Be proactive*: work towards the humane and rational application of EBM.
2. Ensure guidelines are appropriate for local use.
3. Ensure that the status of the guidelines is clear.
4. If the organisation is officially to adopt them ensure that all concerned know this, agree it and have copies.
5. In some instances you may need to ensure that the audit mechanism is engaged to assess the guidelines when they are in use.

Externally

6. Ensure that purchasers understand the general and local limitations on the use of guidelines.
7. Accept guidelines as part of a service specification only if the team involved agree and "let out" clauses are written into the service specification.
8. Ensure that purchasers use EBM equitably adopting not only those guidelines that lead to cheaper care, but also those guidelines that lead to better but more expensive care.
9. With centrally produced guidelines channel responses back to the place from whence they originated (professional group, Royal College, etc) to assist the process of continual modification and updating.
10. Avoid the use of the word *EBM* as a mantra.

The words *EBM* and *audit* have become mantras for managers in hospitals just as "holistic medicine" and "shared care" have for GPs. There is danger that the simple repetition of the word in debate and documents will somehow confirm the worthiness of intent and that writing it in a contract will ensure purity and cheapness. Beware the word. Beware the fashion.

Managed care

We have already seen how doctors have, willingly or otherwise, given up their role of sole determiners of medical care, and we know that their relationships to patients may subsequently have been damaged by what we might call resource-led care, in which the available resource is quantified and the care which doctors are allowed to offer is tailored to that quantity. With the help of EBM and their personal experience and commitment, clinicians may still define what they *believe* to be best for their patients, but may have to accept that circumstances prevent them from *delivering* it. The next stage is potentially more sinister for clinicians and patients. In managed care the individual clinician's role in defining "best" treatment is usurped by the managed care process. Best treatment is then defined by an external group, and protocols based on it are modulated by considerations of cost and resource availability. At its crudest this requires doctors simply to make the diagnosis (and they may even be constrained in how they do this); thereafter the protocol takes over. That is managed care. The historic arrangement whereby the decision about how best to manage patients' illness is decided between clinicians and patients has been invaded by a process defined and managed by others who may or may not themselves be clinicians but who, nevertheless, do not have that primary relationship that doctors have established between themselves and their patients and which has always been judged to be the patient's safeguard. This is an environment where the stakes for doctors, patients, and managers are high in human, professional, and financial terms. In the USA, where about 140 million people are covered by some sort of managed care arrangement, the organisers of managed care are personally and corporately making enormous amounts of money and doctors are having their judgments and their incomes challenged as never before. One might think that

that side of it is not necessarily a risk in the UK, but doctors' abilities to provide what they think best for a particular patient will be eroded and we will need to come to terms with that. There will also be great temptations for future governments to abrogate responsibility for controlling an unmanageable and expensive health service to commercial organisations who will promise to control costs for a fee.

There are a few experiments with managed care in Europe, most emphasising quality and efficiency from patients' perspectives. The French introduced mandatory practice guidelines for a range of 147 common conditions. The guidelines, agreed professionally, were implemented from 1994 to 1995 and a system is in place to fine those who strayed too far from them. The French are not notably acquiescent to bureaucracy, yet a review of the practice of 13 000 doctors led to only 75 of them being fined.[72] One hopes this reflects a close approximation of the guidelines to best clinical practice. Ensuring that the guidelines were written by professional groups not influenced by financial considerations may have been relevant.

It is predicted that managed care will generally be applied more subtly in Europe than it has been in America though it should be noted that enthusiasm for "managed care" is on the wane. But before the new NHS espouses managed care with expected vigour you would do well to read a series of three papers by Fairfield et al in the BMJ.[73,74,75]

To warn yourself of the dangers of managed care in so far as it represents a profit/savings-led approach to health care you could also read "The two cultures and the health care revolution" by McArthur and Moore.[76] These very senior US authors identify 12 potential hazards from the shift to commercial managed care. Some of these are currently only applicable in the USA but others are already apparent in the UK, including downgrading of personnel, gagging clauses, neglect of research, and loss of choice.

The future of managed care

If purely professional considerations about the optimal care of patients are allowed predominance over financial and bureaucratic ones, managed care may merely be the careful application and facilitation of EBM and the smoothing of the process of delivering that care. Not all clinical care will be affected. The role of medical managers will be central to the humanisation of managed care and to ensuring that the hearts and minds of the clinical team are engaged. Clinical managers may need to expend a lot of negotiating effort explaining to purchasers that managed care is a professional exercise undertaken by professionals and not simply a further vehicle for bureaucratisation of the service. This is not a fanciful anxiety. One of the first sets of guidelines which have slipped into managed care (though it is not called that) has been the British Association of Surgical Oncologists' guidelines for the management of breast cancer. Government agencies have now turned this into a blueprint for managed care and are already expending large amounts of their own and others' time and energy in requiring documentation of each tiniest step in the protocol to ensure "compliance".

I used to be a doctor
Now I am a Health Care Provider

I used to practise medicine
Now I function under a managed care system

I used to have patients
Now I have a consumer list

I used to diagnose
Now I am approved for one consultation

I used to treat
Now I wait for authorisation to provide care

I used to have a successful people practice
Now I have a paper failure

I used to spend time listening to my patients
Now I spend time justifying myself to the authorities

I used to have feelings
Now I have an attitude

Now I don't know what I am.

(quoted by Fairfield[77])

6.9 Complaints and litigation

Although we are healthier than we have ever been we are more anxious about our health than any past generation, in addition our old notions of misadventure, Acts of God, and sheer bad luck have been cast aside and replaced by an unmodulated culture of blame. Health is to be perceived as a right, a natural state even, and if we do not remain healthy then someone must be to blame.[78] It is hardly surprising therefore that some patients complain. In fact, the number who do so formally is very, very few even in the current epidemic of complaint. The hospital services receive 28 000 written complaints a year which represents a tiny fraction of the millions of contacts during the year.[79] The small number of complainants, the fact that some of them are readily seen to be merely vexatious, plus the hurt felt by staff when a complaint is received, can lead to a culture of ignoring complaints or at least of not taking them seriously. That is wrong; all the pundits say it is wrong and detailed recommendations and protocols exist for dealing with complaints. More of that later. But first for the sceptic just a moment's reflection on why most of us hate complaints; maybe the better to understand the pattern of our response.

I suspect the great majority of doctors, nurses, and others in the NHS feel that they are doing the best that they can with inadequate resources in difficult circumstances. The patients traditionally shared this ethic as if we were all still in the Blitz together; we did not like it but we would do our best together. The patient who complains that their bed in the air-raid shelter is too lumpy or there is plaster dust in their tea clearly does not share the ethic and when there is personal spite as well, "*You* allowed my bed to get lumpy", "*You* did nothing to stop plaster dust getting in my tea", staff feel doubly aggrieved. I have trivialised the example to make a point. Complainants feel their complaints passionately but the personal consequences for staff involved in a complaint can be very significant. Doctors have killed themselves because of the stress of a long-running complaints process, many others say it is a factor in seeking early retirement. Nurses, clerks, and others simply leave the service. I would say there is one important—very important—message from this. It is this. Every complaint has the capacity not only to inform staff for the purposes of improving the service (the Official view) but also has the capacity to harm, demoralise, and discourage them. The harm is sometimes proportionally many times greater than the complaint would seem to merit. Protocols for handling complaints must reflect this. The current practice of assuming the patient or customer is always right is erroneous in the context of a nationalised health service. Many complaints are ill founded or the errors they report unavoidable. I believe that where the staff involved are not at fault they must be supported and defended. This may even involve defending a case legally at greater cost than simply pretending to be wrong and making a quicker and cheaper settlement. If we cherish our staff as much as our patients we owe them this.

Now that we have got that off our chest, back to the handling of complaints.

The culture of complaint

People have always complained about poor service, we all do it, but the recent rise in the numbers of complaints about health care seems to have coincided with the arrival of "The Patient's Charter" and its successor the more blandly named "NHS Guide". You may, if you wish, view these as the "Great Leap Forward"—a cultural revolution—in so far as it tried to tighten up a perceived, lackadaisical attitude to quality in the public services. A cynic's retort might be that it was simply a way of trying to improve a few, high-profile, measurable items at no cost while shifting the blame for failure in the NHS on to the front-line staff. Both interpretations may be true. What is also true is that centrally devised standards as well as distorting the way health care is delivered mandate patients to complain. The complaints are, interestingly, not just about failures to meet the defined standards, but a whole variety of other issues. The one-way nature of complaints reflects the untrammelled individualism, the *"liberalisme sauvage"* set in motion by Margaret Thatcher, and the increasing mistrust of public institutions and authority in any guise that has followed.

Facing up to complaints

In spite of everything I have said thus far most complaints are genuine and reflect a patient's real unhappiness with what has happened. That unhappiness needs treating and in the process much may be learnt about the defective processes and personalities within the organisation. What should we do? Firstly, try to avoid situations where problems mature into complaints. This requires the people at the scene to render first aid. It needs honesty and forthrightness at the time of a problem and a preparedness to talk it through with the patient.

You may feel that this is a natural response for staff, but it is not reliably so and in our trust we found it necessary to issue a card to all staff (Figure 6.9). This attracted some derision but appears to have had a beneficial effect. Where a complaint has actually been made in writing it should be documented, dealt with through a formal process whose principles were defined by the NHS Complaints Procedures of 1996.[80]

Principles of managing complaints

The NHS complaints procedures are based on the Hospital Complaints Procedure Act 1985, modified in 1996 to obtain certain key objectives:

- ease of access to the system for complaints
- a simple, rapid, open process common to all parts of the NHS
- fairness for complainants and staff alike
- lessons from complaints to be used to improve patient services
- investigation of complaints to be entirely separate from any subsequent disciplinary proceedings.

Informal complaints

Simple comments and complaints are sometimes resolved simply by there being an easy mechanism for making them and allowing the matter to be resolved before it has a chance to fester and become a formal complaint. A readiness to listen, to explain, and to apologise are crucial to resolving matters at this stage. Evasiveness and delay allows the complainant to readily assume a "cover up". It is the Department of Health's intention that most oral complaints should be resolved at the time or within two working days.

Formal complaints

If they are to be acted upon, formal complaints must be made by patients over the age of 16 who have a normal mental capacity, though other people may complain on the patient's behalf with the patient's written authority. In general, complaints must be made within six months of the event complained about or from the moment at which the patient realised there had been a problem. These time limits can exceptionally be extended.

COMPLAINTS INFORMATION CARD

DEALING WITH A COMPLAINANT

- Sort out the problem yourself where you can
- Listen and show interest
- Take the complaint seriously
- Be helpful and understanding
- Find out the nature of the complaint
- Offer an apology and investigate
- Where you cannot immediately help, identify ways to solve the problem
- Where you cannot solve the problem, involve a senior member of staff from your ward/department
- Refer the complainant to the information in the Trust's complaints leaflet

Guy's and St Thomas' Hospital Trust

COMPLAINTS INFORMATION CARD

DEALING WITH A COMPLAINANT

Where you cannot solve the problem do involve a senior member of staff or the Quality Directorate but do not just shuttle the complaint around.

TIME SCALE FOR DEALING WITH COMPLAINTS

- Written complaints must be acknowledged within two days of receipt
- Complaints should be resolved and the complainant have received a full response within 28 days of receipt

Confidentiality

- All patients are entitled to absolute confidentiality
- Staff should limit the discussions of complaints to those staff immediately concerned and treat all complaints as confidential

For help and advice in complaints handling contact:
The Directorate of Quality & Nursing
Guy's Tel 0171 955 4552   St Thomas' Tel 0171 922 8238

Guy's and St Thomas' Hospital Trust

Figure 6.9 Laminated card for staff, reminding them how to deal with complaints.

Essentially, the process of dealing with complaints can go through three quite separate stages.

1. Attempted local resolution.
2. Independent review panel.
3. Appeal to the Health Service Ombudsman.

Local resolution   Every effort must be made to resolve complaints promptly and locally. If the immediate informal response by the person who receives the complaint does not satisfy the complainant then there should be a speedy and open investigation; this is normally undertaken by specially appointed complaints staff skilled in not only laying their hands on the details and interpreting them but also in mediation. Experience shows that 75% of grievances may be resolved promptly in this way if the process is truly open and sympathetic. What must *not* happen is that complainants are dismissed, ignored, or at the very worst, has it implied that a complaint will influence the quality of care that they receive in future. If the complaint is justified someone, ideally a person close to the event, should be prepared to make a proper apology for what has happened. Doctors are often worried about doing this for fear it will imply liability, but it does not. The important thing is that if an apology is due it should be given.

Tensions between the organisation and complainants may be eased by the mediation of a trust's PALS (Patient Advocacy and Liaison Service).

Written complaints must all culminate in a response in writing from the chief executive of the health authority or trust. Some written complaints are multifaceted and require quite careful investigation of the clinical circumstances, obtaining statements from clinicians, and a direct approach to clinicians and other staff to ask their views on what happened. All those responses need to be put together and a reply constructed which the chief executive can then sign and send out to the patient. The Department of Health intends that this should always be completed within a month. That sounds a long time and it probably seems so for complainants, but it is exceptionally difficult to assemble the notes of a complicated case and the views of clinicians, whom we have noted earlier will be disheartened and/or irritated by the complaint. It is important to remember that the regulations require that any response that refers to matters of clinical judgment must be agreed by the practitioner before it is sent out.

If complainants are dissatisfied with the outcome of "local resolution" to an oral or written complaint, then they may request an independent review.

Independent review   If a complainant asks for an independent review that does not invariably entitle them to have such a review. Reviews are difficult and time consuming and it is critical that requests for them are properly assessed. Regulations allow this in so far as they are first looked at by a "convenor". This will be a non-executive or lay director of the trust or health authority. It is a difficult task. The convenor, who by definition has no medical knowledge, has to try to obtain a comprehensive picture of what has happened, not only in relation to the events themselves but also to find out whether the local resolution procedures were properly carried through. In doing this the convenor may need to take independent advice, usually clinical from outside or inside the trust or health authority. The convenor must discover whether legal proceedings are actually underway or threatened. At the end of this assessment the convenor may decide that:

- the local resolution process needs more time and effort put into it and is worth pursuing further
- the local resolution adequately answered the complaint and that there are no grounds for proceeding to an independent review
- a review should not proceed because legal proceedings are underway
- an independent review should be undertaken.

For an independent review a "panel" is set up with a lay chairperson who is chosen from a regional list held by the Secretary of State. The panel consists of three people:

- the chairperson
- the convenor
- another lay person.

The chairperson has the discretion about how the panel goes about its business but is required to arrange things within the following rules.

1. The proceedings must be confidential.
2. The panel must have access to all records about the handling of the complaint so far.
3. If the complaint is clinically based the panel must have access to the relevant part of the clinical record.
4. The panel must give the complainant and the practitioner complained against a reasonable opportunity to express their views in writing or verbally.
5. The panel should not operate in a confrontational or legalistic way, as its intention is solely to establish the facts. No legal representation of any party is allowed.
6. Complainants may be accompanied by an adviser, for example, from PALS. Similarly, practitioners may be accompanied by a representative from their professional organisation or other "friends". Advisers and friends may only contribute to the proceedings with the approval of the chairperson.

Once the panel has accumulated the information about the case it must, if it relates to clinical matters, appoint at least two external independent assessors. These assessors in turn will have access to all the records and may interview or even examine the patient. They do not then write a report, they merely submit their observations to the lay panel.

When all the facts and the clinical opinions have been gathered, the panel is required to produce a final report, a copy of which is sent to the complainant, the practitioners concerned, and the chief executive. The chief executive will then decide whether any action needs to be taken and advise the complainant of their decision. He/she is additionally required to advise the complainant that if they are still dissatisfied they may take their grievance to the Health Service Ombudsman. All this should take no more than three months, a timescale which is often difficult to meet.

Once the panel has produced its report that stage of the process has been completed and cannot be repeated. The only avenue open to the continuing complainant is the Ombudsman or the law.

Appeal to the Health Service Ombudsman If complainants have exhausted the local resolution and independent review process and still feels unsatisfied, they can appeal to the Health Service

Ombudsman, more properly known as the Health Service Commissioner. The Ombudsman will review all the paperwork which has been generated by the local resolution and independent review processes and may appoint his own independent advice. If the matter is related to clinical judgment, then he/she is required to have the assistance of two specialist assessors. If the Ombudsman decides to go ahead one of their staff will interview the party involved and, in due course, produce a final report which must be sent to the chief executive of the organisation involved for action, for comments or for recommendations. The Ombudsman may also make their own recommendations about disciplinary action in relation to clinicians and other practitioners or may suggest that a reference is made to the GMC or other regulatory body. The Ombudsman does not, him- or herself, have any disciplinary powers.

It is important for clinicians to understand that they also have the right of appeal to the Ombudsman if they feel that the local resolution or, more likely, the independent review process has led to them "suffering hardship or injustice", and obviously in any such appeal they would want to seek the assistance of their medical defence organisation.

Problems with the system

Although the new complaints system seems straightforward and equable to all parties, there has been much dissatisfaction with it, particularly in relation to the independent review stage. Those who have experienced it have not infrequently reported that the panel has been unsympathetic, confrontational, and sometimes straightforwardly aggressive, or that it has led to the initiation of disciplinary procedures against staff or their suspension without "due process". Even though these problems seem to arise from the overreliance on lay persons for coming to a judgment (and one would think it would make it more likely that claimants would be satisfied), evidence is that they are frequently not satisfied by the panel process if it does not go in their favour. A Consumers Association study reported to the Commons Select Committee on Health in 1997 found 40% of complainants were unhappy with the way their complaint was dealt with.

The NHS Trust Federation has reviewed the workings of the new process and has not found evidence of difficulty in meeting the timescales. Anxieties have been expressed about the difficulty of recruiting non-executive directors to be assessors or to participate in panels. The whole business of the panel was found to be too time consuming, too bureaucratic, and had no way of dealing with vexatious complainants. Plans are, however, afoot to radically overhaul the review process though no changes to legislation have yet occurred. See http://www.doh.gov.uk/complaints/reform.htm.

Mediation

It would be nice to believe that mediation in some form or another could resolve many of these issues, particularly as they are said so often to concern patients or their relatives simply wanting to find out what went wrong. Litigation is inherently confrontational and a bad and a slow route to resolution. Mediation, however, has not yet found a place in the system but I have inserted it here before litigation in the faint hope that it might be used more. If you are interested there is helpful information about it on the National Health Service Litigation Authority (NHSLA) website (http://www.nhsla.com).

Complaints that turn into litigation

However carefully you deal with complaints the outcome often seems to be unsatisfactory for complainants rarely fall on the complaints officers' necks thanking them for resolving the problem. The complainant who only wants to find out what happened may be content simply with the information, but the aggrieved complainant often wants more and the mollifying tone of the letter from the complaints officer or chief executive who acts as an intermediary between those involved and the complainant may be the very agent that further irritates the complainant who becomes more angry rather than less. Such complainants may not even understand their own motives; for example, when the complainant is the relative of someone who has died the complaint may be an expression of the anger of grief inappropriately expressed. Not infrequently the complainant wants not an explanation but somehow to punish the system for a real or imaginary hurt sustained. A sanitised apology does not suffice, they want floggings, heads on poles, long periods of incarceration in dank dungeons with rats. But these are no longer open to them, so embittered complainants pass from process to process, from complaints officer to panel, to Ombudsman, to their MPs and then eventually to law, using up inordinate amounts of staff time and emotional energy. This may be a happy reflection on the options of the population to pursue a just solution but it is a very unwelcome process for most hospitals.

Some complainants go straight to a solicitor without even stopping off to make a verbal complaint in the hospital. Whatever the route, the endpoint of threatened or actual litigation is important for the institution. The costs, both of defending or of losing a case, will fall on the institution and such claims are rising and form a significant part of the budget. Between 1995 and 2000 clinical negligence claims rose sevenfold to a total value of £2·6 billion; by 2002 the figure had risen to £4·4 billion. Single claims can be enormous, and in the context of the NHS may be an inappropriate way to spend the nation's resources. Brain damaged babies account for 80% of outstanding claims by value and 26% by number. A brain-damaged baby judged to be so because of defective hospital care can take several million pounds out of the NHS budget and yet the state still needs to care for the child. A child similarly brain damaged by some other misadventure is similarly cared for but receives nothing. Litigation lawyers remind us that claims are not about to reach a ceiling in terms of absolute numbers. It has been said that only one in 12 of those who have a good case for litigation actually proceed. This is obviously a source of distress to lawyers who see missed opportunities for enrichment, but it has helped to keep down the overall cost to the NHS.

The reasons why most complaints do not go to law is probably nothing to do with the success of the internal complaints, but simply the difficulties of it. Going to law is almost solely the privilege of the legally aided. Access to legal aid is quite easy for those whom a means test finds eligible. The decision as to whether to grant legal aid is based on the advice of applicants' lawyers who have, of course, a direct financial interest in advancing the claim and tend to take little expert medical advice before putting forward the case for legal aid. The numbers of personal injury cases supported by legal aid have thus risen by a factor of four over the last 10 years. A measure of the excessive ease with which legal aid is obtained in medical negligence cases is the low success rate of such actions. The

Woolf Report noted that only 17% of the 12 576 legally aided medical negligence cases closed in the year to 1st April 1996 were successful. The success rate in cases for other forms of personal injury such as accidents at work is 85–90%. The whole process is very protracted, the average time from the issue of proceedings to conclusion is six years and five months.

Medical managers should be aware of three changes that will affect practice.

1. Conditional or contingency fees ("no win, no fee").
2. The recommendations of the Woolf Report.
3. Changes in the regulations relating to the granting of legal aid.

No win, no fee

The legislation to allow lawyers and their clients to come to conditional agreements about fees—the fee being conditional on the outcome of the case—came into effect in July 1995. There was alarm that this would allow the "ambulance chasing" and speculative litigation common in the USA to appear in the UK. Fortunately, there are other differences in the law between the UK and the USA that make this unlikely. In the USA the plaintiff and the defendant pay their own costs regardless of the outcome, whereas in the UK the loser must pay the other party's costs. The option, therefore, of not having to pay your lawyer if you lose does not guarantee a risk-free exercise for the plaintiff, although in theory it is possible to *insure* for the other party's costs if you lose, the uncertain outcomes of medical litigation can make this prohibitively expensive. The no win, no fee arrangement also puts greater pressure on the plaintiff's solicitor to check that the case is worth pursuing, and that pressure is much greater than it is in legally aided cases. Overall, the system will probably reduce rather than increase the number of vexatious and speculative claims.[81] Doctors in the UK also retain the continuing privilege of the application of the "Bolam Test". The Bolam Test is applied by a judge to claims that a doctor was negligent and requires him to accept a defence that a responsible body of practitioners trained in the same speciality would have acted similarly,[82,83] although the Bolitho Case of 1997, if cited in future, could require that medical experts' views as well as reflecting sound medical practice must demonstrate that they have considered the comparative risks and benefits of any action.[68]

The Woolf Report

The Woolf Report[84] reviewed the whole of the civil justice system in England and Wales and recommended radical change. Medical negligence litigation did not escape his attentions because he considered most cases currently to be unduly long, complex, and expensive. In a sample of medical negligence cases that his commission reviewed they found the average time from first contact with a lawyer to resolution was 65 months, and for claims worth less than £12 500 the legal costs of just one side averaged 137% of the claim's value. Lord Woolf also found that unmeritorious cases were pursued for too long and the degree of lack of cooperation and mutual suspicion was greater than in any other class of litigation.[85]

The recommendations of the report have been summarised as follows.

1. Greater effort at prevention and early resolution of disputes. As steps towards this he recommended that medical record keeping should be better, the procedures for local resolution of problems should be clearer and that there should be more use of mediation with jointly instructed experts where possible and a greater use of experts' meetings. Overall though he recommended a more sparing use of experts.
2. An improved summary disposal procedure to weed out weak claims and weak defences.
3. The introduction of a system of plaintiff "offers to settle" with sanctions where a defendant unreasonably refused to cooperate.
4. Claims of £10 000 or less to be handled by a slimmed-down procedure with a limited range of legal processes conforming to tightly controlled timetables and costs.
5. Large and complex claims to be handled by a "multitrack" process where the management of each case legally is decided by the courts themselves rather than by lawyers.

Much of this was welcomed although there is considerable scepticism about the prospect of only a single medical expert being involved in some cases. The final outcome of the Woolf Report is yet to be determined but it would be prudent for medical managers to follow the arguments and the alternative proposals through as they evolve.[86] Despite efforts to reform by the year 2000 the costs of settling claims of less than £50 000 still exceeded damages in 65% of cases.

In the meantime, in response to Executive Letter (96)11, which outlines policy for handling clinical negligence and personal injury litigation, most NHS organisations should have established a clear set of rules within their organisation.

Changes to legal aid legislation

The costs of legal aid are rising annually and are a headache for the government. Recent changes to the rules so as to reduce access to legal aid excluded medical negligence cases. Even though seven years had elapsed the Lord Chancellor's Legal Services Commission in 2002 was still having to press legal firms to screen cases more critically before applying for legal aid using the same standards as they would use for no win, no fee cases. When seen from clinical managers' viewpoint there have really been very few perceptible changes since the Woolf Report and they should therefore live in the continued expectation of protracted, frustrating, and often futile combat with the legal advisers of the legally aided.

A brief and useful summary to complaint and litigation handling may be found in *Clinical Negligence and Complaints: a clinician's guide.*[87]

References

1 Barnes P. Managing change. In: Simpson J, Smith I, eds. *Management for Doctors*. London: BMJ Publishing Group, 1995, pp 45–53.
2 Webb AK, Hanley SP. The conflict in transferring a cystic fibrosis specialist service between two hospitals in Manchester. *BMJ* 1997;**315**:1009–11.
3. Fulop N, Protopsaltis G, Hutchings A *et al.* Process and Impact of Mergers in the NHS. *BMJ* 2002;**325**:246–7.
4 Goddard M, Ferguson B. *Mergers in the NHS*. London: Nuffield Trust, 1997, p. 85.
5 Kennedy I *et al.* Dear Mr Dobson. *BMJ* 1997;**315**:147.
6 Klein R. The Case Against. *BMJ* 1996;**314**:503.
7 Thornton S. The case of Child B—reflections of a chief executive. *BMJ* 1997;**314**:1838–9.
8 Klein R. Priorities and rationing. Pragmatism or principles? *BMJ* 1995;**311**: 761–2.

9 Smith R. Rationing health care. Moving the debate forwards. *BMJ* 1996;
   312:1553–4.
10 Ham C, Honigsbaum F, Thompson D. Priority setting for health care. In:
   Oakley A, Williams AS, eds. *This Politics of the Welfare State*. London: UCL
   Press, 1994, pp 98–126.
11 Smith R. Being creative about rationing. *BMJ* 1996;**312**:391–2.
12 Weale. Rationing health care. *BMJ* 1998;**316**:410.
13 Welch HG, Mogielnicki J. Presumed benefit: Lessons from the American
   experience with marrow transplantation for breast cancer. *BMJ*
   2002;**324**:1088–92.
14 Gillam S, Penceon D. Managing demand in general practice. *BMJ* 1998;
   316:1895–8.
15 Wyatt JC. Hospital information management. The need for clinical
   leadership. *BMJ* 1995;**311**:175–80.
16 Audit Commission. *For Your Information: a study of information
   management in the acute hospital*. London: HMSO, 1995.
17 Lock C. What value do computers provide to the NHS hospitals. *BMJ*
   1996;**312**:1407–10.
18 Benson T. Why general practitioners use computers and hospital doctors
   do not. *BMJ* 2002;**325**:1086–93.
19 Furedi F. *Culture of Fear: risk taking and the morality of low expectation*.
   London: Cassell, 1997.
20 Leape L. Cited in *BMJ* 1997;**315**:970.
21 National Audit Office. *Health and Safety in NHS Acute Hospital Trusts in
   England*. London: HMSO, 1996.
22 Ennis M, Vincent CA. Obstetric accidents; a review of 64 cases. *BMJ*
   1990;**300**:1365.
23 Soljak M. Volume of procedures and outcome of treatment. *BMJ*
   2002;**325**:787–8.
24 Vincent C, Clements. Clinical risk management—why do we need it?
   Clinical Risk 1995;**1**:1–4.
25 Reason JT, Carthey J, de Leval MR. Vulnerable System Syndrome. *Qual
   Health Care* 2001;**10**(Suppl 2):1121–5.
26 Hiatt HH, Barnes BA, Brennan I *et al*. The study of medical injury and
   medical malpractice; an overview. *New Engl J Med* 1989;**321**:40.
27 Wilson RM, Runciman WB *et al*. The quality in Australian Health Care
   Study. *Med J Aust* 1995;**163**:458–71.
28 Editorial. *JAMA* 1998;**279**:1200.
29 Pickersgill T. The European working time directive for doctors in training.
   BMJ 2001;**323**:1266–7.
30 Gordon F. Editorial. *Clin Med*. JRCPL 2002;**2**:41–2.
31 Wilson JA. The impact of shift patterns on healthcare professionals.
   J Nursing Management 2002;**10**:211–19.
32 Aitken M, Paice E. Trainees' attitudes to shift work dependent on grade
   and specialty. *BMJ* 2003;**326**:48.
33 Weed LL. New connections between medical knowledge and patient care.
   BMJ 1997;**315**:231–5.
34 National Audit Office. *Clinical Audit in England*. London: HMSO, 1995.
35 Gnanalingam J, Gnanalingam MG, Gnanalingham KG *et al*. An audit of
   audits: are we completing the cycle? *J R Soc Med* 2001;**94**:288–9.
36 O'Brien T *et al*. Audit and feedback: effects on professional practice and
   health care outcomes. *Cochrane Database Syst Rev*. 2000;(2):CD000259.
37 Pollock A, Evans M. *Surgical Audit*. London: Butterworth, 1989.
38 McErlain-Burns TL, Thomson R. The lack of integration of clinical audit
   and the maintenance of medical dominance within British hospital
   trusts. *J Eval Clin Pract* 1999;**5**:323–3.

39 Miles A *et al.* Clinical Audit in the NHS: fact of fiction? 1996;2:29–35.
40 Farrell L. Audit my shorts. *BMJ* 1995;**311**:1171.
41 Editorial. *J R Coll Phys* 1996;**30**:415–25.
42 Lord J, Littlejohns P. Evaluating healthcare policies: the case of clinical audit. *BMJ* 1997;**315**:668–72.
43 Fletcher DR. Laparoscopic cholecystectomy: what national benefits have been achieved and at what cost? *Med J Aust* 1995;**163**:535–8.
44 Johnson A. Laparoscopic surgery. *Lancet* 1997;**349**:631–5.
45 Womack C, Roger S, Lavin M. Disclosure of clinical audit records in law: risk and possible defences. *BMJ* 1996;**315**:1369–70.
46 Rangachari J. Evidence based medicine: old French wine with a new Canadian label. *J R Soc Med* 1997;**90**:280–4.
47 Sackett DL. Evidence Based Medicine. What it is and what it isn't. *BMJ* 1996;**312**:71–2.
48 Appleby J, Walshe K, Ham C. Acting on Evidence. *NAHAT Research Paper* 17, 1996.
49 NHS Centre for Reviews and Dissemination. *Effective Health Care* 1996;2(8).
50 Muir Gray JA. Evidence based, locally owned, patient centred guideline development. *Br J Surg* 1997;**84**:1636–7.
51 Grimshaw JM, Russell IT. Effect of clinical guidelines on medical practice. *Lancet* 1993;**342**:1317–22.
52 Naylor CD. Meta-analysis and the meta-epidemiology of clinical research. *BMJ* 1997;**315**:617–19.
53 Green J, Britten N. Qualitative research and EBM. *BMJ* 1998;**316**:1230–2.
54 Knottnerus JA, Dinant GJ. Medicine based evidence, a prerequisite for evidence based medicine. *BMJ* 1997;**315**:1109–10.
55 Smith GD, Egger M. Meta-analysis. Unresolved issues and further developments. *BMJ* 1998;**316**:221–5.
56 Egger M *et al.* Bias in meta-analysis detected by a simple, graphical test. *BMJ* 1997;**315**:629–34.
57 Egger M, Smith GD, Phillips AN. Meta-analysis. Principles and procedures. *BMJ* 1997;**315**:1533–7.
58 Gøtzsche PC. Why we need a broad perspective on meta-analysis. *BMJ* 2000; **321**:585–6.
59 Le Lorier J *et al.* Discrepancies between Meta-Analyses and Subsequent Large Randomized Controlled Trials. *New Engl J Med* 1997;**337**:536–42.
60 Editorial. *Lancet* 1992;**339**:1197–8.
61 Editorial. *Lancet* 1997;**350**:675.
62 Swales J. The troublesome search for evidence: three cultures in need of integration. *J R Soc Med* 2000;**93**:402–7.
63 Haynes BR, Devereaux PJ, Guyatt GH. Physicians and patients choices in evidence based practice. *BMJ* 2002;**324**:1350.
64 Tracey JM *et al.* The validity of general practitioners' self assessment of knowledge: cross sectional study. *BMJ* 1997;**315**:1426–8.
65 Platt R. *Private and Controversial.* London: Cassell, 1972, p. 124.
66 Kerridge I *et al.* Ethics and evidence based medicine. *BMJ* 1998;**316**:1151.
67 Sackett DL. EBM what it is and what it is not. *BMJ* 1996;**312**:71–2.
68 Bolitho v City and Hackney Health Authority. *The Times Law Report,* 27 November 1997.
69 Tingle JH. Do guidelines have legal implications? *Arch Dis Child* 2002;**86**:387–8.
70 Grol R. Beliefs and evidence in changing clinical practice. *BMJ* 1997;**315**:418–21.
71 NHS Centre for Reviews and Dissemination. Getting Evidence into Practice. *Effective Healthcare* 1999;**5**:1–14. (Available at http://www.york.ac.uk/inst/crd)

72 Durand-Zaleski I, Colin C, Blum-Boisgard C. An attempt to save money by using mandatory practice guidelines in France. *BMJ* 1997;**315**:943–6.

73 Fairfield G *et al.* Managed Care: Origins, Principles and Evolution. *BMJ* 1997;**314**:1823–6.

74 Fairfield G *et al.* Managed Care: Implications of Managed Care for Health Systems, Clinicians and Patients. *BMJ* 1997;**314**:1895–8.

75 Fairfield G *et al.* Managed Care: Disease Management. *BMJ* 1997;**315**:50–3.

76 McArthur, Moore. The two cultures and the health care revolution. *JAMA* 1997;**277**:985–9.

77 Quoted by Fairfield G. *BMJ* 1997;**314**:1896.

78 Porter R. *The Greatest Benefit to Mankind: a medical history of humanity.* London: HarperCollins, 1997.

79 Department of Health. *An Organisation with Memory.* London: The Stationary Office, 2000.

80 Department of Health. *Complaints—listening ... acting ... improving: Guidance on implementation of the NHS complaints procedure.* London: DoH, 1996.

81 Barton A. Conditional fees: access to justice for all. *Clinical Risk* 1997;**3**:130–1.

82 Jones MA. *Medical Negligence,* 2nd edn. London: Sweet & Maxwell, 1996.

83 Baird RN. The vascular patient as litigant. *Ann R Coll Surg Engl* 1996;**78**(Suppl):278–87.

84 Lord Woolf. *Access to Justice.* London: HMSO, 1996. (Available at http://www.lcd.gov.uk/civil/final/contents.htm)

85 Lord Woolf. Changing landscapes in medical negligence. *Clinical Risk* 1997;**3**:202–4.

86 Lord Otton. A three-stage scheme for medical negligence. *J R Soc Med* 1998;**91**:421–6.

87 Green A, McConnachie K. *Clinical Negligence and Complaints: a clinician's guide.* London: Royal Society of Medicine Press, 2002.

7: The future

7.1 The future of medical management

Predicting the future is a dangerous business because most predictions end up wrong, but in the matter of the future world of medical managers I think we can see a fair way ahead. Indeed, if they are about to take off, flight crews ought to be able to see to the end of the runway at least.

Medical management will survive

It is reasonable to ask whether clinicians will continue to be involved in management in the future. It is prudent to ask why they might not wish to continue. One reason for withdrawal would be as a consequence of the general change in the attitude of doctors to service. There are many factors altering the relationship of doctors with their job and with their patients, of which the interference of the state is only one. Changes in hours, lack of continuity, defensiveness formalised in risk management, and a general lack of societal feeling all contribute. Doctors have always committed a lot to medicine and for most it is the all engaging passion of their lives and that is one of the things that leads them into the peripheral commitments of research, publishing, committee work and, more recently, management. Current training programmes will one presumes deliver future consultants who are younger and more narrowly trained into posts that are more specialist and more driven by protocol and *diktat* than is the case now. Such doctors will need the stimulus of variability in their careers and time in a managerial post will surely form one of the options for "career development" for them. By contrast, if the combination of general social change and a continuing interposition of non-clinical agencies between doctors and their work continues, they may increasingly become less altruistic, less vocational, more nine to fivers, and less willing to take on extra work. Altruism in a non-religious society requires reciprocity of support and respect between patients and doctors. Heedlessly eroded by politicians and the media that reciprocity is failing.[1] We are already noting some difficulties in recruiting doctors into management posts as the first waves step down. In my experience the reasons for this are many, but they boil down to the hassles, inappropriate managerial targets, the conflict of loyalties, and lastly, an unwillingness for most of them to become involved in those parts of management which are not really related to patient care. Of course they could always be bribed back by the right payment but that would be the wrong reason for their involvement. This is a gloomy scenario and my preferred prediction is that their natural streaks of leadership and curiosity will continue to ensure the recruitment of doctors into management.

The medical managers of the future

The roles of medical managers as currently practised have in general evolved or been defined on the basis of historical experience. We can expect the role to evolve further in the future as experience grows and clinicians who have "gone into management" build on their experience better to define the roles of their successors. The majority of those successors will need to be not just clinicians co-opted to give credibility and support to the management process, but will need to be separate animals. I suggest that most will not want to spend their time worrying about the details of finance and personnel, negotiating of contracts, and monitoring compliance, nor will they wish just to be clinical governance police. They will want their involvement to be primarily, perhaps even exclusively, in the areas which non-clinical managers cannot so easily understand: quality and performance, education, and the strategy for delineating optimal care and the needs of patients. *Doctors should do what only doctors can do.*

So there will be clinicians in management. What may preoccupy them? Let me guess at the following.

1. *Everything thus far described in this book*: I doubt if any of the difficulties to do with making teams work, adapting to limited resources, clinical governance, improving quality, and performance will disappear.

2. *Accountability* and a changed view of *professionalism*.
3. *Scientism* versus *humanism*.
4. *Education.*
5. *The shape and style of the NHS.*

There are, of course, other things that will preoccupy them as doctors. The growth of team working, the march of technology, the tide of information and how to handle it, the shift into primary care if there is to be one, or perhaps the shift back from primary care into secondary care. Who knows, but these are general concerns of doctors and this book is about medical management.

7.2 Accountability

It is said that we are now in the third health revolution. The first was the arrival of technology to improve care, the second the impact of financial constraints, the third the era of accountability.[2] The pressure for accountability could in the future see medical care going in one of two directions: either deprofessionalised, overregulated, overaudited, a further slip into a morass of bureaucracy; or it could adopt a new respect for redefined professionalism where doctors, nurses and others are trusted to deliver the best care they can in the circumstances, the whole process being constructively monitored and reviewed as distinct from policed. Doctors in management, if they remain primarily doctors and keep their nerve, will be well positioned to catalyse these latter changes.[3] Politicians, the media, and the public, as well as other professionals, will need to accept that professionalism is something to be cherished, not subverted. Doctors, like other professionals, will need to maintain their pride in being professionals, keep a positive grip on it. To quote Peter Hennessy:

> for years I have nurtured a speculation that future scholars might see in eighties and nineties Britain a malign factor at work—loss of nerve about those activities and institutions in which we could still claim to be truly worldclass. ... The crumbling of our self-confidence as a professional society has led to breaches appearing in our institutional walls through which has marched an assertive army, management consultants, accountants and self-proclaimed reformers who

evangelically recite the latest acronymic babble ... My embryonic thesis about institutional nerve loss ... depicts its beneficiaries as "The Three Horsemen of the Contemporary Apocalypse; Money, Management and Marketing". All three, as they ride in brandishing their crude performance indicators, are quite incapable of appreciating that ... the whole is greater than the sum of the parts; that's the point of institutions—we do together what we cannot do alone. The eighties and nineties have seen the thoughts of those who actually do the work written off as "producer views" which must be discounted, as they are driven by vested interest. And, sadly, there were enough genuine inefficiencies and restrictive practices to give the managerialists a case. But all too often you had the sense that the reformers disliked, even despised, the objects of their zeal— thinking that, at best, they needed saving from themselves and, at worse, they required punishing for past under-performance.[4]

That was not written about medicine and the NHS but it applies to that institution as closely as it does to those to which it referred.

These threats are not temporary ones. They leave with us a legacy of a third force in our institutions, an increasingly powerful group of people who do not carry out any of the core functions but merely monitor, analyse, hypothesise, and direct. They have too vested a personal interest to be easily displaced and like so many computer viruses become an integral if unhelpful part of the operation of the machine. A new generation of doctors may come to regard them as a natural feature of a landscape and be untroubled by them. But to be thus untroubled they will need to know them and their ways well and cooperate or confound them as is appropriate. This sounds like an echo of the antimanagerialism deprecated in Chapter 1 of this book, but it is not. It is a desire to keep as much of the decision making in health care as close to those who carry out the work as possible, and that means those who have daily contact with patients, that is, clinicians, nurses, and other professionals, for I believe only these people can truly concentrate on what the patients need and want. Nevertheless, if doctors are going to go on claiming that right of primacy then they will need to polish up their act as far as patients are concerned. *Clean* up their act you might say and this means not taking the relationship with patients too much for granted. It means working harder to prove that they can be trusted to do the best for the patient. The list of issues arising

> **Box 7.1 Issues of clinical governance raised by the Bristol cardiothoracic surgery case and identified by the GMC**
>
> - The need for clearly understood clinical standards
> - How clinical competence and technical expertise are assessed and evaluated
> - Who carries the responsibility in team-based care
> - The training of doctors in advanced procedures
> - How to approach the so-called learning curve of doctors undertaking established procedures
> - The reliability and validity of the data used to monitor doctors' personal performance
> - The use of medical and clinical audit
> - The appreciation of the importance of factors, other than purely clinical ones, that can affect clinical judgment, performance, and outcome
> - The responsibility of consultants to take appropriate actions in response to concerns about their performance
> - The factors which appear to discourage openness and frankness about doctors' personal performance
> - How doctors explain risks to patients
> - The ways in which people concerned about patient safety can make their concerns known
> - The need for doctors to take prompt action at an early stage where a colleague is in difficulty, in order to offer the best chance of avoiding damage to patients and the colleague, and of putting things right
>
> (Reproduced from *GMC News*, 1998.)

from the Bristol case identified by the GMC (Box 7.1) is a good checklist for any doctor or manager wishing to approach this issue formally.

The NHS at present has the huge virtue that it allows patients to believe that doctors and others within it are not doing things to them or for them simply for financial gain. Nevertheless, if we consider the darker sides of twenty-first century Western society, the culture of complaint and the rise of selfish and individualistic consumerism, the doctor–patient relationship can become positively adversarial. Medical managers can do as much as anyone to keep the relationship on the rails. At present it sometimes seems that the expected way that doctor–patient relationships will be improved is through formal education of staff. There is a great danger that in pursuing that end the educational theorists advising the GMC and the medical schools will over-egg the curriculum—insisting on early and formal training in ethics, social, and legal issues. I am not convinced that the full legal and ethical curriculum proposed by a consensus group of clinicians, philosophers, lawyers, and theologians and put out as "non-negotiable"[5] will really do what is needed. The authors have presumably not seen how easy it is to "turn off" undergraduates and trainees by heavy handed formal education in these topics. By contrast medical managers, with undergraduate and postgraduate tutors, can ensure that these topics are drip-fed into all trainees through the medium of communications, seminars, audit meetings, and committee agendas throughout their training so the issues are seen in context.

Trust

In establishing accountability and redefining professionalism, part of the deal which professionals need to make with the public goes beyond tightening up professional competence and self regulation. It involves (and this is the bit the management books forget to mention) somehow reassuring patients that doctors are still on their side while not concealing the constraints. Doctors who have been medical managers will, one hopes, desist from the unfortunate habit that many non-managerial clinicians have, of negatively emphasising to patients the resource problems, saying how awful politicians, the Department of Health, and managers are. Mature clinicians need to explain the difficulties while making it clear to patients that they remain on their side. In this the doctors' role is no different from when they are treating diseases. When faced with a patient with a new diagnosis of cancer of the bronchus, one hopes most clinicians do not launch into a denigration of the fickleness of God, the venality of tobacco manufacturers, the shocking lack of a screening programme, and the slowness of the referring GP. The clinician focuses on what can be achieved for the patient.

The patients and those who plan and manage the NHS may need to learn that performance can probably not be improved endlessly and error certainly cannot be wholly obviated by yet more micromanagement. Indeed, these may make things worse. The habit of trust will have to be relearnt.

7.3 Scientism versus humanism

This was ever a problem for doctors. Technology, the military arm of science, always carries risk to patients as well as benefits, particularly when it articulates the habit of action in preference to reflection. EBM, managed care, and protocols facilitated by computers will be even more culturally dominant in the lives of doctors soon, extending the tentacles of scientific truism further into the soft corners of medical art. In our fixation on their benefits we may lose the subtleties that distinguish the profession of medicine from the professions of engineering or of physics. It is not just that we may lose humanity but we may also lose some subtlety of perception—"the concept is always the enemy of intuition".[6] By identifying the disease and by automatically translating it into a protocol, we potentially lose our ability to see the patient, just as when we call a thrush a thrush, or a willow a willow, we may cease to see the bird or the tree for its true self.

But enough of this namby pamby stuff.

The hard area of EBM will be its imposition or otherwise in day-to-day care. Swales, in his essay on "Culture and medicine"[7] stressed the importance of realising that health involves more than "scientism" (the belief that science-based evidence can resolve all the difficulties of the health service). He reminds us that we cannot extrapolate scientific absolutism to the relativism of cultural values, that society is heterogeneous, that individuals have different assessments of what they want, and what they will tolerate. Wyatt went further by stressing the need for going beyond "explicit knowledge" that is the territory of EBM and its acolytes into the realms of "tacit knowledge", which is that personal, case by case intuitive knowledge that clinicians interpose between patients and mindless obedience to explicit knowledge. To codify that tacit knowledge so that it becomes available other than in the simple context of team working is the new challenge.[8] In their role as go-betweens, between managerialism and patients, medical managers need to develop their role as arbiters in the imposition of an increasingly structured set of rules about what should be done to whom, by whom, when, and at what cost. They may be the focal point of debate about care which bounces back and forth between what *can* be done, what the protocol says *should* be done, and what *ought* to be done for this particular patient. Establishing themselves as the people within the organisation who have the right to make those judgments may be more difficult. As go-betweens medical managers also need to grapple with a shift from a service-led (you get what we provide) to a needs-led (you get what you say you want) service, which is the consumerist face of a more patient-orientated service. One of the great stimuli to team working should be that it will refine these professionally human judgments and also give them more clout.

7.4 Education

Education you may say is not the business of medical managers but if they are to intercede between the patient-focused world of clinicians and the resource-focused world of managers, they need to educate both parties, not in a sense of formal lectures but the continuing education of giving facts, putting views, and changing attitudes and behaviour. In her paper on changes in continuing medical education, Angela Towle summarised the responsiveness needed of medical education as follows.

- Teach scientific behaviour as well as scientific facts.
- Promote the use of information technology.
- Adapt to the change in doctor–patient relationship.
- Help future doctors to shape and adapt to change.
- Promote multiprofessional team working and care.
- Help future doctors handle broader responsibilities.
- Reflect the changing pattern of disease and healthcare delivery.
- Involve health service employers and users.

It is difficult to envisage a situation where medical managers are not prime participants in that sort of educational process.[9]

Medical managers may also find themselves embroiled in radical change in the eduction of SHOs and SpRs. The government currently seems determined radically to change the way this is done so as to speed it up and produce doctors tailored to speciality needs. Gone will be the prolonged broad education, the cosy habits of apprenticeship, the searching examinations. Instead, there will be defined and targeted education interrupted by regular way points where trainees' competence is formally assessed. Much more of consultants' time will need to be explicitly dedicated to this process with serious implications for service delivery. Much paperwork will be generated. Consultant status will be achieved much earlier and postCCST training will need to occur. Issues of competence, procedure licensing, and supervision will regularly occur and medical managers will be responsible for ensuring that during all this continuing upheaval the ship continues to follow a steady course.

7.5 The shape and style of the NHS

The hospital as an institution has come to dominate the NHS; since its inception their share of the budget rising from 54% in 1948 to 70% by the mid-1970s. The main thrust of the trend to involve doctors in management has come within hospitals, which one might think lend themselves to being manageable units easily managed. However, it has—as this book has intimated—been very difficult and is only just achieving a fragile existence as a working system. Yet some suggest that the future of the NHS lies in deconstructing its current arrangements and developing new ones where teams link up across traditional boundaries to provide a host of integrated care networks. It all sounds persuasive and worthy, but little is written about how such systems might be managed in a day-to-day way and by whom. If this is to be the shape of the future health service we will need to define how primary care and hospitals will manage the processes that can deliver seamlessly managed patterns of care.

When the new government was elected in 1997 the phraseology of documents about the NHS changed. There was less talk of competition and cost and marketing. New headlines were about cooperation and equity and the White Paper of December 1997, *The New NHS: Modern and Dependable*, seemed to be heading in the right direction but with a new flush of quangos, promises of more money yet running through it still the old controlling reflex, mixed with the socialist instinct to make everything the same. Blair built on the Thatcherite legacy of challenging large interest groups (miners in her case, professionals of all sorts in his) and gave us *The NHS Plan*. This is heroic in scope but the conceptual basis of the NHS remains sacrosanct. The NHS is still to be centrally funded and centrally managed, but the plan as well as delivering more money delivered objectives too large, too complex, and too explicit to be shrugged off as the fault of front-line workers when they are not achieved.[10,11] Top down planning like this has enormous risks and even the government accepts that there is a "do or die" element to *The NHS Plan*. If it cannot deliver the volume and quality that is called for, despite providing the same funding as more effective health providers elsewhere in the developed world, the basic concept of the NHS may become untenable;[12,13,14] indeed, it might simply sink under the weight of its own superstructure.

We live in interesting times and new medical managers who want a feel for the swirls and countercurrents of what is going on can be confidently recommended to read Rudolf Klein, *The New Politics of the NHS*,[15] to find out how we got to where we are and Harrison and Dixon, *The NHS Facing the Future*[16] to see where we might go.

In the meantime we are told that what the public wants is convenience, quality, and explicitness. If the government will fund it and the medical profession engage properly in the management of its delivery then there is no reason why the public should not get what it wants and have it provided by a re-energised medical profession.

References

1 Jones R. Declining altruism in medicine. *BMJ* 2002;**324**:624–5.
2 Relman AS. Assessment and accountability. *New Engl J Med* 1988;**319**:1220–2.
3 Medical Professionalism Project. Medical professionalism in the new millennium: a physicians' charter. *Lancet* 2002;**359**:520–2.
4 Hennessy P. Book review of "Utopia and Other Places" by Sir Richard Eyre. *The Independent,* 22 January, 1997.
5 Doyal N, Gillon R. Medical ethics and law as a core subject in medical education. *BMJ* 1998;**316**:1623–4.
6 Roose-Evans J. *Inner Journey, Outer Journey.* London: Darton, Longman, Todd, 1998, p. 185.
7 Swales J. Culture and medicine. *J R Soc Med* 1998;**91**:118–26.
8 Wyatt JC. Management of explicit and tacit knowledge. *J R Soc Med* 2001; **94**:6–9.

9   Towle A. Changes in healthcare and continuing medical education for the 21st century. *BMJ* 1998;**316**:301–4.
10 Allen I. Challenges to the health services: the professions. *BMJ* 2000; **320**:1533–5.
11 Cunningham D. The NHS Plan and Clinicians. *Clin Med JRCPL* 2002; **2**:134–8.
12 Eyres J, Dewar S. Delivering the NHS Plan: a case of 'constrained innovation'. *Health Care UK 2001*. London: King's Fund, 2002, pp 34–40.
13 Timmins N. After the NHS Plan, what next? *Health Care UK 2001*. London: King's Fund, 2002, pp 82–4.
14 Curley A, McClure G, Spence D, Craig S. The new NHS: modern, definable? *Clinician in Management* 2002;**11**:15–23.
15 Klein R. *The New Politics of the NHS*, 4th Edition. London: Pearson, 2001.
16 Harrison A, Dixon J. *The NHS Facing the Future*. London: King's Fund, 2000.

Index

Page numbers in **bold** refer to figures; those in *italics* refer to tables or boxed material.